So you want to Registered Care Home Manager?

Your questions answered about <u>becoming</u> a home manager AND practical tips on <u>how to run a compliant home</u>

Liam Palmer

Copyright © 2020 Liam Palmer

All rights reserved, including the right to reproduce this book, or portions thereof in any form. No part of this text may be reproduced, transmitted, downloaded, decompiled, reverse engineered, or stored, in any form or introduced into any information storage and retrieval system, in any form or by any means, whether electronic or mechanical without the express written permission of the author.

ISBN: 9798682073481

PublishNation
www.publishnation.co.uk

Dedication

This book is dedicated to Warren Canicon,
Sam Griffiths and Claire Childs.
I still remember your kindness.

Contents

Foreword by Dr Umesh Prabhu 7
Introduction by Tim Dallinger 9
About the Author 11
1. Legal Responsibilities of the Care Home Manager 13
   1.1 The CQC – the Care Quality Commission 13
   1.2 Safeguarding 16
   1.3 Health and Safety for residential care 18
2. Care Management Responsibilities 23
   2.1 Care Quality Essentials 23
   2.2 Clinical Support Tips for Care Home Managers 28
3. General Management Responsibilities 41
   3.1 Care Home Recruitment – how to get it right 41
   3.2 Managing Finance 44
   3.3 The Importance of Audits 49
   3.4 Managing the Rota 51
   3.5 How to Manage the Night team in Residential Care 52
   3.6 Meetings 53
   3.7 Complaints and compliments 54
   3.8 The Importance of Confidentiality 55
4. Q & A 59
5. Bonus Material! 83
   5.1 Secrets of Winning that New Care Job or Progression 83
   5.2 Five Tips On How To Improve Your Care Home 87
Index 95
A Final Note from the Author 97

Foreword by Dr Umesh Prabhu

I first met Liam on the professional network LinkedIn. Liam interviewed me about culture and leadership for his podcast "Care Quality – meet the leaders and innovators" in July 2019 and a further episode on patient safety in October 2019. Liam and I have met many times since that initial meeting. We have a shared passion for the impact of good quality on care outcomes for those who use care services.

The largest group of users of residential care are older people, those who are 85+. Over the next 20 years, this group is due to grow significantly due to the baby boom generation ageing. This age group can be very vulnerable – often managing multiple health conditions and/or dementia. In order to ensure this vulnerable group of people are well cared for, we need a new generation of leaders to run the new care homes appearing across the UK.

This book will help senior carers, deputies and current home managers develop the specific skills required to run a care home effectively. So much of the focus in healthcare is about compliance – this is crucial but the missing ingredients for sustainable compliance are the leadership and management skills that underpin it.

I welcome this book. I gather it is Liam's third on doing what he can to raise standards across residential care by sharing good practice in management and leadership as a home manager and leadership expert. It is no small thing to commit the hours required to make this level of contribution to this overlooked area of healthcare. It reflects his belief that managers with well-developed management skills can run care services more effectively.

In my experience as an NHS Director, I found that by setting and modelling high standards as a leader, we were able to improve culture, morale, and crucially quality outcomes. It is the least understood part of healthcare – that good culture, good leadership = good quality, safe healthcare.

Liam is an authoritative voice in the residential care sector with a deep understanding of this dynamic with a passion for developing and upskilling new managers. As a resource to further this end, I commend this book to you.

Dr Umesh Prabhu, NHS Medical Director – Bury (1998 - 2003) and Wigan (2010-2017)

Introduction by Tim Dallinger

It is my pleasure to provide an introduction to this book, *So you want to be a CQC Registered Care Home Manager?* As a care home provider myself and a social care consultant for the last 12 years, I know that the managerial skills of the home manager are an important determinant of whether the service is well run and, by default therefore, whether the service is run in a way that the CQC will regard as compliant with good care.

With standards of care compliance becoming more rigorous, and with the media's often negative portrayal of residential care, the job of registered manager is becoming even more demanding. The main route to become a care home manager in the UK is through relevant experience and completing the CQC/skills for care recommended qualification pathway – the QCF level 5 Diploma in Leadership in Health and Social Care. There is much merit in this broad qualification but there are also skill and knowledge gaps. Liam covered some of these gaps in his book *Leadership secrets for Care Home Managers*. In this very practical follow up, he focuses on how to do the job – whether pressure sores, continence or assessments, he shares the gritty important stuff that all managers need to know to manage their services well.

Liam and I are quite different; I discovered this when he interviewed me for his "Leaders and Innovators" podcast series in September 2019. One of our shared jokes is how long he takes to write something. However, this is because he approaches his work like a piece of art; whether written work or a podcast, he takes time to draw out the true meaning of something and won't let up until it's clear. I think this rigour, applied to the knowledge and skills gaps for a home manager, has led to useful, original content. I have no doubt it will help aspiring managers to make the transition to a senior management role.

Tim Dallinger
Director of Social Care Consultants Ltd

About the Author

Liam Palmer has many years' experience as a care home manager, across a range of providers and facilities. He is keen to share his findings, in the hope of helping to improve quality of care across the board. This is his third book on care home leadership.

What follows is not exhaustive, as certain elements below vary by provider, type and size of service. Your local CQC Inspector and your Local Authority social work/care team may have unique positions on some of these points. What follows is based on Liam's work at mid-to-large homes for older people over the last seven years (2014 – 2020).

Disclaimer – This work is dated 15.07.20 and is a qualified introduction to these matters – it should not be used as a definitive guide to running a home or be considered an actual recommendation. Please ensure you follow the advice on the CQC website, together with the company policies and guidelines from your employer. The views expressed are those of the author.

1. Legal Responsibilities of the Care Home Manager

1.1 The CQC – the Care Quality Commission

The Care Quality Commission is the independent regulator of health and social care in Britain. To manage a care home, you must first be registered with the CQC as "the registered manager" and go through that process, as per Q & A, at the end. Furthermore, the provider and the specific home must already have been registered with the CQC.

CQC Ratings – KLOEs

As the manager of a care home, you will need to have a good working knowledge of the KLOEs – key lines of enquiry. These pose the five following questions: whether a service is considered to be "safe", "effective", "caring", "responsive" and "well-led". These are the CQC standards used to inspect and assess every home. From these inspections come the four ratings, which are: "inadequate", "requires improvement", "good" and "outstanding."

There is a rating given under each of the five KLOEs at the point of rating – an inspection will conclude with a rating for each question and an overall rating for the home. If there are two or more KLOE ratings of "requires improvement", the service is rated as "requires improvement" overall; if there are two or more KLOE ratings of "inadequate", then the service is rated as "inadequate" overall. To be rated as "outstanding" overall, the service must achieve at least two KLOE ratings of "outstanding", with no KLOE being rated as "requires improvement". The overall rating is the measure that determines how the home is regarded in terms of compliance, which in turn reflects (and has an effect on) reputation/public image.

If the overall rating is "good" and above – it is compliant. Residents have a right to care that meets the CQC standards.

In brief:

- **"Inadequate"** – serious breaches, it could lead to the home being closed if the provider doesn't take urgent action.
- **"Requires improvement"** – some breaches, which warrant closer scrutiny. In the inspector's view, the service is below the minimum standard of "good."
- **"Good"** – meets CQC standards. Following inspection, the service is considered to meet the needs of the residents when considering the five KLOEs framework.
- **"Outstanding"** – 3% of services get this, and the rating includes an element of continuous improvement. This is the ultimate rating. All progressive services will aim for this, though there are more "outstanding" ratings in smaller homes. (Often these services are able to be more person-centred than larger homes.)

Most of the time, the ratings are fair and representative of the experience of the residents and the inspector's observations on the day. Sometimes, though, they may be unconsciously biased. This could be based on previous experiences with the home. Sometimes inspections come as expected after the receipt of a PIR (Provider Information Return). In August 2019, the CQC announced that care providers would be required to complete an annual PIR on the anniversary of their first inspection visit. This means that a service rated as "good" or "outstanding" may complete more than one PIR before an inspection visit from the CQC. It also means that the service will no longer get notice that an unannounced inspection is due.

At other times, unannounced inspections come in response to a whistleblower making allegations. The CQC collects data from other sources, often meeting monthly to review homes that are struggling. That way, it can prioritise homes where there are mounting concerns. In some cases, staff can misuse these processes to harm, by giving a false report to the CQC. Most of the time, when these allegations are investigated, they are shown to be unproven and malicious. This is common. If there is an unannounced inspection to check where a concern is raised and it leads to an overall downgrading of the rating to "requires improvement", this is a serious matter. There is a mechanism to challenge an unfair rating as well as unfair comments but most of the time this isn't necessary, as the concern will already have been discounted.

A key point to remember is that the overall CQC rating is also a marker for the public of how well the home is doing. If it is "good" or "outstanding", this gives a positive message to families and, therefore, for admissions. If it is graded as, "requires improvement", it can negatively affect both. This can be difficult if the CQC doesn't come back to check progress for an entire year, as the negative rating will stand for the whole of that time.

I feel that, with the pressures from above via a regional director (in larger organisations) or the owner in smaller organisations, home managers can become overly focused on the inspection rating. The CQC is visiting to check there is quality care in the home, with sound governance and a well-managed staff team, and that all relevant controls are in place. In my view, the primary focus for the home manager should be that the residents experience high-quality care *every day*. In this way, when the inspector comes, there should be nothing to fear from an inspection. The audit schedule and previous whole home audits and accompanying action plans should help protect the home manager from many surprises!

CQC notifications

Registered Managers have an obligation to report various matters and incidents to the CQC – see the whole list of these on the CQC website (https://www.cqc.org.uk/guidance-providers/adult-social-care#notifications).

Two of the most common CQC notifications used as a home manager are:
• Regulation 16 - reporting a death - "the death of a person using the service";
• Regulation 18 – reporting of "Alleged or actual abuse, DOLs (Deprivation of Liberty Safeguards) applied for, serious injuries and incidents reported to the police".
Failing to provide such notifications is considered a serious breach of regulations. The registered manager doesn't need to provide the notifications themselves, but they must ensure that, if the job is delegated, it is completed to the required standard and sent off promptly. A failure to submit a notification to the CQC will result in a rating for the "well-led" KLOE of "requires improvement" (at best).

1.2 Safeguarding

Registered managers have a legal obligation to notify the safeguarding team within their local authority when there has been abuse, suspected abuse, or when a person has been at risk of harm or abuse. The Care Act 2014 changed the definition of a "vulnerable adult" to a "person at risk". A person is "at risk" if they are being harmed or abused, or are at risk of harm or abuse and they cannot protect themselves from it. The abuse can take myriad forms – financial, emotional, physical, psychological, etc. The safeguarding team will decide if it meets their threshold for abuse for a safeguarding alert to be raised formally, leading to further investigation.

Each local authority will have different thresholds. Some with a low threshold will want everything reported. Others will have a higher threshold and use their reporting system only for exceptional or serious ongoing concerns. Suspected abuse also needs to be reported into the CQC using the relevant notifications – Regulation 18. The registered manager (or their representative in the home) needs to speak to the safeguarding team, ask for advice, and then follow this advice. This is an actual, legal obligation.

Good practice with managing safeguarding alerts will usually entail taking immediate action to reduce/eliminate the risk to residents.

After checking with the safeguarding team, it is often necessary to conduct interviews/statements. If the care home is requested to undertake an investigation, it is vital that the person doing this is trained and competent to do so.

By not following the correct procedures – asking "why" questions rather than "what" questions – or interviewing people in the wrong order (alleged victim first, witnesses next, other people next, alleged perpetrator last), the investigation can be ruined.

Generally speaking, there should be a factual investigation to start with, in which all relevant witnesses are interviewed and asked, "What?", "When?", "Where?" and "Who?". The alleged perpetrator should then be questioned regarding the witness statements, to establish their side of events and to verify if it is likely these events took place. The investigating officer would usually do a summary of their findings and pass it to the home manager to review. The home manager would then review the documentation and decide what appropriate action to take – formal or informal, drawing on their own expertise, and the policies of the home/organisation.

Throughout the process, it is the registered manager's job:

- to summarise and discuss;
- to take action and use the case as a learning experience, to ensure it doesn't happen again;
- to listen and show an understanding of the experience of the resident;
- to communicate to the resident what is being done at different points in the investigative process.

In this way, the registered manager is letting the alleged victim feel they've been taken seriously and that serious concerns are addressed appropriately, with due confidentiality. This is a complex area, but these general principles hold.

The key tip is that the registered manager needs to demonstrate a responsible and proactive attitude to deal with these matters – but seek advice from the safeguarding team first. If the manager fails to do this, the safeguarding team may get more closely involved to ensure things are dealt with robustly and effectively.

1.3 Health and Safety for residential care (*see also 2.2: 'Clinical Support Tips for Care Home Managers' and 2.1.1: 'The Delicate Balance of Bed Occupancy versus Residents' Needs'*)

This is a very broad area which is now regulated by the CQC. It was previously overseen by the HSE (the Health and Safety Executive). It is important that registered managers have adequate knowledge of the subject. Often, registered managers will do an IOSH (Institute of Occupational Safety and Health) "Managing Safely" Level 3 day-course and a CIEH (Chartered Institute of Environmental Health) Occupational Health and Safety Level 3 course, to better understand their specific responsibilities. The HSE publishes an extremely useful guide, **HSG220:** *Health and safety in care homes*. This can be downloaded free of charge from the website: http://www.hse.gov.uk/pUbns/priced/hsg220.pdf. The guide is packed with vital information and contains a checklist. Registered managers would be wise to audit their service against this guidance.

Maintaining your building:

Infrastructure: It is vital to keep records which show that the building is professionally maintained, with suitable checks for all plant infrastructure – e.g. gas, electric, water, cookers, lifts, heating and fire doors. Fire alarms must be tested, and service contracts must be up-to-date. The building must be shown to be in a reasonable state of repair.

Equipment: Your records must show that specific equipment in the building is being suitably maintained, e.g. hoists, wheelchairs, slings and bed rails. See the LOLER (Lifting Operations and Lifting Equipment Regulations), and the PUWER (Provision and Use of Work Equipment Regulations), etc. These relate to lifting equipment and any other equipment used in a workplace. Remember that anything used in the course of the work is regarded as equipment and this must be safe and fit for purpose. We have all used a chair instead of a stepladder to change a lightbulb, but in a workplace it is a legal requirement that the correct equipment be used for the task. In this case, even the stepladder needs to meet certain criteria. Another example of poor practice is to use a wheelchair to transport bags of waste out to the bins; this is hazardous practice from the perspective of both safety and infection control.

Furniture: Sofas, beds, and any other furniture being used in the home must be proven to be fit for purpose and safe, with an appropriate quality/design. All materials must be fire-retardant (as per The Regulatory Reform (Fire Safety) Order 2005). The safety of the electrical system needs to be tested and all portable electronic equipment requires PAT testing – this includes portable appliances which belong to service users and staff.

Infection and harm control: You must demonstrate that flooring, sinks and walls are being suitably maintained to avoid risk of harm/infection, as bacteria can accumulate in broken tiles or fittings. The Department of Health published a Code of Practice on the prevention and control of infection in 2013; this provides guidance on how social care providers can comply with their legal responsibilities.

Some requirements include:

- appointing a designated infection control lead;
- writing an annual infection control compliance statement;
- the correct use of cleaning schedules.
- An evidence file is needed to demonstrate controls are in place, including daily/weekly/monthly audits, according to the service and its respective needs.
- Other points include having an up-to-date list of keys, plus holding spare keys for every bedroom (crucial for safety/fire).

Fire Safety: This is a crucial area that needs continual attention. Fire safety needs to be taken seriously by the whole team, and the registered manager needs to provide leadership here. Naturally, there must be suitable alarms in place, and these need to be checked and signed off. There needs to be evidence provided that fire drills are being performed regularly. Door closers need testing and checking. Residents' doors need to be fire retardant to protect the hallway and to provide a period of safe protection from potential fires surrounding each room. The roofing and layout of the building needs to be fit for purpose in regard to fire safety.

Good practice with managing fire safety is to carry out frequent full fire drills at different times of the day/night/weekend. This ensures all staff members understand their responsibilities and will know what to do in the event of an actual fire and how to document this clearly. Good practice would likely show where there are gaps in training or knowledge and what is being done to address them. This process provides evidence that the service is being managed appropriately, complying with the relevant health and safety legislation.

PEEPS: A personal emergency evacuation plan (PEEPS) will state who is in the building and how they need to be evacuated in the event of a fire. Night-time staffing levels need to reflect these needs. This must be updated whenever there is an admission/discharge.

Business Continuity Plan: The Business Continuity Plan offers contingency planning for devastating events – e.g. catastrophic fire, flood, etc. These possible events require some consideration – for instance, if the building was on fire, where would the residents go? This needs documenting in advance. Whilst this may seem like a lot of paperwork (it is!), once it is done properly, it simply needs reviewing yearly. You never know when you may need this. When dealing with the lives of vulnerable people in your care, don't take unnecessary risks. Contingency planning and clear, up-to date-documentation are how we manage those risks.

The safe storing of food, beverages and certain medications

Temperatures for fridges and freezers are both significant areas within health and safety because, if the temperature is not optimal/consistent, it can impact on the characteristics and safety of any food, beverages and medication held there. Fridge temperatures should be in the range

1°C - 8°C and a temperature of 3°C is ideal. Chilled food *must* be kept below 8°C and if food is delivered, then the delivery temperature should be below this. Frozen food deliveries must be below -18°C and freezers should also operate below -18°C. Temperature control of hot food is of course equally important. Often care homes prepare food too far in advance and then there are issues of keeping it warm. You can hot hold food for a maximum of two hours and it must be kept above 63°C.

For food: Poor temperature control can make the food unsafe to eat, even leading to possible food poisoning. It is essential to adhere to rules around stock rotation and the keeping of food with clear dates. There is often confusion around "use by", "best before" and "display until" dates. "Best before" means exactly that: it is at its *best before* that date and is safe to eat *after* that date, although the longer the food is kept, the poorer its quality will be. It is illegal to sell or serve food past midnight on the date specified on the "use by" date label. It is also vital to maintain separate shelves in the fridge and different chopping boards for different foodstuffs. Meat, for example, needs to be stored separately from vegetables, etc.

There are further protocols to reduce the risk of contamination and therefore food poisoning. This includes not reheating cooked food more than once. Remember that cook-chill products, such as ready meals or pre-prepared foods as used in some care homes, have been cooked once already in the factory. So, when you cook this food, you are actually reheating it. The principles are stricter than in an individual's home but, when dealing with elderly or physically vulnerable residents, safety through reducing risk is an important consideration.

For medications: Poor temperature control can mean that any medicines kept in the fridge lose their effectiveness and are no longer safe to be used. This could be through temperatures being too low or too high. Stock control is also important – whatever is out-of-date needs to be disposed of appropriately.

The importance of good housekeeping practices
Cleaning routines must be followed, using the correct products. The correct products need to be safely stored away from residents. These practices need to be audited as evidence that the registered manager is fulfilling their health and safety obligations. See COSHH (Control of Substances Hazardous to Health Regulations) and risk assessments.

Dangers of the kitchen for vulnerable people
This pertains to the importance of security around access to sharp knives, detergent, cookers, hot water or even foods (e.g. it could be dangerous if a person with severe diabetes consumes an excess of sugary snacks). Whilst this level of control over the environment may seem excessive, bear in mind that a person with a severe learning difficulty or mid-to-later stage dementia may have no sense of place or risk regarding these things. The home manager has a legal obligation to take measures to keep everyone safe using various controls under the Health and Safety at Work Act 1974. The risk assessment processes and documentation is the way these risks are managed. These need to be adhered to, documented clearly, and reviewed periodically.

2. Care Management Responsibilities

2.1 Care Quality Essentials – what you need to know about doing assessments, care plans and managing incidents and accidents

2.1.1 The Delicate Balance of Bed Occupancy vs. Residents' Needs: Resident need and dependency versus occupancy

For the safe and sustainable running of your home, it is crucial to consider the levels of resident need and dependency. This is about managing risk and workload, in order to manage the well-being of those in your care. In general, you will have a staffing ladder for your home – this is usually a sliding scale of resident numbers versus staffing hours. There is usually the desired number and then the minimum safe number. For example, you may be scheduled to have six staff members on shift (ideal); five staff would be the minimum safe level. Four would be unsafe. Needs will vary so, when you have a combination of residents requiring exceptional levels of support, you may not be able to safely run the floor with fewer than six. For a floor with 20 residents, you may have a budget for three carers on shift in the morning and three in the afternoon. This equates to a ratio of 6.7 carers to 1 resident (20/3). Balancing the levels of resident need with staffing levels and the budget is an important skill.

Risks of high level of need in the home: As discussed earlier (*see also 3.4: 'Managing the Rota'*), staffing ratios are only part of the story. It is also about how strong your staff teams are (depth of experience and care knowledge/mix of hard-workers/team spirit /how well they know the residents/length of service can all be factors). You need to know your residents and staff team well. It's a judgement call. The care team will always want residents who are generally easier, and so they will complain whatever you do, but you need to understand what their actual capacity is. Give them enough to be manageably busy, and increase their confidence by building the resident population carefully and thoughtfully.

Balancing needs with bed occupancy pressures: If several residents pass away, there will be pressure to rebuild occupancy. If the residents referred to you have high dependency, what do you do? If you take them all, the owner/regional director may be happy temporarily – but if, later, there is an increase in falls and complaints, and staff start leaving because of an unmanageable workload, it could be that some of those admissions were not well-thought-through. The registered manager position is the responsible one. You need to weigh all things up and make good decisions for the home, residents, families, teams – and for those who oversee and audit the service.

When you can't meet the need: If, when you do an assessment, after careful consideration and liaising with your team, you conclude that you can't meet the need, you must simply state this, briefly explaining why. Sometimes social workers and hospital discharge teams under pressure will try to influence you to clear the bed/take the person, even if you have declined. They may disagree with your reason for not accepting the resident. You need to be aware of the constraints across the social care system – be courteous and professional but, as RM, do right by your home and by your residents. This is your legal obligation. The owner/home, the families, the residents and the regulator are all trusting you to do the right thing.

In the end, you need to run a service that has a good reputation, that staff are happy to work for, that manages risks responsibly and has a profile of resident that you can care for with skill. If you manage quality well, in time, the reputation of the service will mean you will get referrals and fill the home. Never underestimate the power of reputation for your care home. Treat every person you come into contact with as a customer, to be treated with respect and courtesy, and you won't go far wrong.

2.1.2 Assessments for potential new residents/assessing levels of support required

Your needs assessment for potential new residents will determine whether or not you can meet their needs. Different companies use different assessment templates. It's important a standard form is used, to ensure you compare those you assess objectively, and so you get skilled in using it. Most assessment templates have a scoring system.

I use the Barthel Index. I look for potential new residents who score within the "low rating" and stick to that. As my care home becomes more established and the skills-mix of the team changes, I may take some residents with greater needs (medium rating), on a case-by-case basis.

Assessments need to be especially clear on certain important considerations – a person's level of mobility, any serious risks or allergies, any recent surgery or serious health conditions that need managing, special dietary needs, current medication – particularly any strong medication to manage conditions. Also, family details – next of kin, previous GP's surgery, date of birth and NHS number are all needed. You have to keep in mind that, if a resident moves into your care home and becomes poorly enough to pass away, you would need enough detailed information to manage this appropriately. Particular care needs to be taken regarding their wishes, who to contact, etc. Do they have a current-and-signed Do Not Resuscitate (DNAR) order in place? It all matters.

2.1.3 The Care Plan

Care plans are the home manager's roadmap and control document to enact the resident's wishes, needs and wants, demonstrating they are respected. The details will come from the assessment document. When your resident moves in, the fundamental needs within the care plan need acting upon. Different organisations have different protocols – but a rule of thumb is that, within 48-72 hours of admission, you need to have an operational, sufficiently-detailed care plan in place. Some organisations have respite care plans (a more concise version) for shorter stays.

Good care plan practice will include the following:

Using person-centred language. For example, consider the statement: "I enjoy cereals/toast for breakfast and occasionally love to have a cooked breakfast – no beans", versus the less personal: "He has a good appetite/likes any type of breakfast food." This differentiation is significant, as it helps the carers to see the person, to have a sense of the resident expressing preferences, and it also offers the idea that, over time, their preferences may change and the care plan will need to evolve and reflect this. The term "person centred" is more than just about using someone's name; it is honouring their individuality and getting the care service to adapt to that individuality as much as is practically possible.

Regular care reviews with the resident – in some cases, this is monthly; in others, quarterly. This review can be held with the resident alone, sometimes with family as well, sometimes with a person appointed with power of attorney (POA) for care for that individual. There is a balance to be struck here. What is not good is a situation in which all the sections of the review are simply signed without due regard. There should be a proper conversation, to ensure all aspects of care delivery are fit for purpose and to note and respond to any changes or other preferences. The key point is that, as a resident's needs change, this must be reflected in the care plan and care delivery. Failing to do this can be a breach of the CQC guidelines around "safe", "caring", "effective and "responsive." For example, if a resident came to the home using a stick and now occasionally needs a wheelchair to get to the dining room, this must be covered in the care plan. Risk assessments *must* be reviewed, too. I met with the outgoing Chief Inspector of the CQC a couple of times, and she made it very clear that the "voice" of the service user/resident should be at the heart of all care. The views of the recipients of care must be solicited, considered and acted upon and documented accordingly.

Care plans – paper versus electronic: In much of social care, there is a marked distrust of electronic care plans. There is a strange commitment to paper plans and the use of paper for record-keeping, which is practical but archaic. The argument for paper records is that having one record in your hand is a great way of keeping track of care, but the downside is significant – lots of repetition, duplication and time taken away from residents through the writing up of records. I believe the wariness around electronic care plans is based on reviewing care plan technology from about 10 years ago. These were simply desktop versions of paper care plans. I think the distrust was merited at the time (I did a project on offerings available in 2018). However, the next generation of care software is mobile/PDA driven, intuitive (icons in place of words to capture activity) and well-designed to manage risks, including alerts for changes in condition. Two of the leading brands of care monitoring are **Person Centred Software (PCS) and Nourish**.

If a care home uses electronic care plans, the benefits need to be explained, and staff need to be consistent in their use of them. The CQC is positive about the adoption of tech where it is used consistently and is fit for purpose. After personally running many residential services, I believe the primary benefit of well-designed care planning software is about managing risks – if something adverse is happening, there is an alert (paper plans don't do this). The secondary level of benefits includes: ease of access, ease of update and ease of accessing/sharing info on a resident in an organised and consistent way (subject to usual GDPR guidelines of good practice).

2.1.4 Dealing with incidents/accidents

It is essential to capture potentially significant occurrences mainly involving residents (though occasionally staff) that will be reviewed, with possible further actions taken to demonstrate good and effective care. It also puts into context if there are further complications with an individual – it can help to demonstrate a build-up of occurrences, e.g. for a person with declining mobility, they may start to slip or fall more, or a change of medication may lead to more falls. Recording these means action will be taken and family will be informed. These are my basics of first principles around what to record.

Next, you need to agree the specific definition of an "incident" or "accident" within your organisation and team. What is the threshold? This is not being pedantic; it is an important aspect of your home governance. Some homes will define an "accident" as anything causing actual harm (a skin tear) or something more significant. The threshold needs to be clear and used consistently. Some homes see "incidents" as occurrences that didn't cause any harm. For example, residents who have hit their head will often be monitored for the next 24 hours and have their well-being recorded every two hours to note any change – while other, high-risk, residents who hit their head will be admitted to hospital as a precaution immediately after, as per agreement with their doctor/care plan.

The other important part of this is the loop – there needs to be a loop of reviewing, checking, monitoring and signing off if any action needs to be taken before closing the incident investigation. This is a tool used in care homes to ensure residents are kept safe and that the registered manager is evidencing that they are providing safe and effective care for those they support. There will also be a monthly analysis, showing the times of falls (any patterns), the location of falls, etc. This is helpful info; for example, there may be more falls at handover if the handover takes too long with the whole team in attendance. The management data will reveal this and action *must* be taken and documented in response to these findings.

2.2 Clinical Support Tips for Care Home Managers

2.2.1 Medication Management – what you need to know as registered manager/home manager

Medication is a huge area of compliance within a care home. Therefore this paragraph can only provide a snapshot of "how to" for the registered manager. Please visit the link provided: http://www.nice.org.uk/guidance/sc/SC1.jsp

The importance of following NICE guidelines: It is advised that every care home manager is fully up-to-date with the care home medication policy, along with the NICE guidelines for "Managing medicines in care homes" in order to understand what is required in the area of medication administration and management. Be aware that, over time, the guidelines may be updated and, under the home manager's duty of care, it is important to update oneself on a regular basis.

Checks to make with staff around medication management:

- Ensure that all staff members who administer medication are up to date with the correct level of medication training.
- Ensure that all staff delivering medication understand the process.
- Ensure that all staff administering medication receive regular competency testing, including in the intervals between formal training.
- Ensure that all medication-trained staff know how to order medications and what day to place an order for medication so that residents do not run out.
- Ensure that all medication-trained staff know how to receive, store and dispose of medication safely.
- Ensure that all medication-trained staff know how to support residents who self-administer their medicine.
- Ensure that medication administration charts are filled in correctly with the correct codes.
- It is useful for medication-trained staff to sit in on medication reviews with community staff.

Use the Six Rights of Medication!

Be aware of and conversant with the Six Rights of Medication. Ensure that the staff in the care home are familiar with them and can in time recite and understand them:

1 Right client;

2 Right route;

3 Right drug;

4 Right dose;

5 Right time;

6 Right documentation.

Other considerations around best practice/reducing risk with medication management:

- Consider spot-checking staff on the Six Rights: this can easily be carried out on a walk around the home.
- Consider, as the care home manager, whether it might be useful to complete an advanced level medication course yourself, as many do.
- Consider appointing a medication champion.
- Carry out regular audits, part audits and full audits covering all shifts over all days – you cannot audit medication administration enough.
- Utilise any pharmacy professionals that may be located within the wider organisation, or consider getting to know the local clinical commissioning team's pharmacist, as they can be a great source of support and help.
- Only buy in good-quality medication training.
- Use NICE resources : Care home staff administering medicines: https://pathways.niceorg.uk/pathways/managing-medicines-in-care-homes/care-home-staff-administering-medicines.pdf
- Know and share the guidance from the CQC for providers with regard to controlled drugs: https://www.cqc.org.uk/guidance-providers/adult-social-care/storing-controlled-drugs-care-homes

2.2.2 Continence Care – what you need to know as registered manager

Continence care is paramount within a care home, because it reduces healthcare-related harm and promotes the well-being of the resident; it also preserves dignity by showing that value is placed upon the person and their needs. It is essential that the care home manager is fully aware of the needs of their residents and has sufficient depth of knowledge about good practice with continence care to manage those needs effectively.

Firstly, let's get a better understanding of incontinence before we explain good practice in managing the symptoms:

Urinary incontinence is more common than an inability to control bowel movements. Urinary incontinence is also more common in older people, especially women. Such incontinence can often be cured or controlled.

What causes incontinence of the bowels?

Injury to the nerves that sense stool in the rectum or those that control the anal sphincter can lead to faecal incontinence. The nerve damage can be caused by childbirth, constant straining uring bowel movements, spinal cord injury or stroke.

What are the risks for urinary incontinence? How are they categorised?

For older women, if they have previously been through pelvic surgery, pregnancy and childbirth, these are major risk factors, as is menopause. Types of urinary incontinence include: stress incontinence, overflow incontinence, urge incontinence or an overactive bladder, functional incontinence, mixed incontinence, total incontinence and bed-wetting.

What happens in the body to cause bladder control problems?

(See: https://www.nia.nih.gov/health/bladder-health-older-adults) The body stores urine in the bladder. During urination, muscles in the bladder tighten to move urine into a tube called the urethra. At the same time, the muscles around the urethra relax and let the urine pass out of the body. When the muscles in and around the bladder don't work the way they should, urine can leak. Incontinence typically occurs if the muscles relax without warning.

What are the causes of urinary incontinence?

Incontinence can happen for many reasons, such as: urinary tract infections (https://www.niddk.nih.gov/health-information/urologic-diseases/bladder-infection-uti-in-adults?dkrd=hiscr0045), vaginal infection or irritation, or constipation (https://www.nia.nih.gov/health/concerned-about-constipation). Some medicines can cause bladder control problems that last a short time.

When incontinence lasts longer, it may be due to:

- Weak bladder muscles;
- Overactive bladder muscles;
- Weak pelvic floor muscles;
- Damage to nerves that control the bladder from diseases such as multiple sclerosis, diabetes (https://www.nia.nih.gov/health/diabetes-older-people), or Parkinson's disease (https://www.nia.nih.gov/health/parkinsons-disease);
- Blockage from an enlarged prostate (https://www.nia.nih.gov/health/prostate-problems);
- Diseases such as arthritis (https://www.niams.nih.gov/health-topics/arthritis) that may make it difficult to get to the bathroom in time;
- Pelvic organ prolapse, which is when pelvic organs (such as the bladder, rectum, or uterus) shift out of their normal place into the vagina. When pelvic organs are out of place, the bladder and urethra are not able to work normally, which may cause urine to leak.

How does incontinence affect men?

Most male incontinence is related to the prostate gland. Causes include:

- Prostatitis—a painful inflammation of the prostate gland;
- Injury, or damage to nerves or muscles from surgery;
- An enlarged prostate gland, which can lead to Benign Prostate Hyperplasia (BPH), a condition where the prostate grows as men age (https://www.nia.nih.gov/health/prostate-problems#problems).

Is Incontinence linked to dementia?

Urinary incontinence, or unintentional urination, is common in people who have dementia. It can range from mild leaking to unintentional urination. Less commonly, it also refers to unintentional bowel movements, or faecal incontinence. Incontinence is a symptom that develops in the later stages of dementia. Between 60 – 70% of those with Alzheimer's will go on to suffer from incontinence issues.

Incontinence aids

The following aids are available: pads, pull-up pants, male continence sheaths, bed pads, waterproof mattress protectors and catheters.

What is involved in good continence care?

Good continence care involves having the right aid for the right person, with costs managed appropriately. The following points will help you provide good-quality continence care:

Pads: ensure that all staff know and understand that residents who are prescribed pads as part of their continence care need to wear the right product at all times, i.e. **light flow, heavy flow, day and night pads.** By doing so, you are promoting dignity and independence, reducing the chances of overflow and spillage, and promoting comfort.

Ensure that staff have been trained in the correct level of continence care, and in particular understand the different types of pads, sizes and times of day for which they are intended/needed, i.e. day or night pads.

If a resident uses a catheter, ensure that the care plan is up to date and is followed to the exact letter. Ensure that all staff understand and have been trained in catheter care according to their level of responsibility, i.e. nursing or residential home.

Audit the care plan regularly to ensure that staff members are following it as directed.

Ensure that the contact details for specialist staff and advice are available to all staff. If an assessment is required, there is usually a clinical nurse specialist in the community who can make a referral for continence support if necessary. This may differ in areas of the UK, depending on the location of the home.

Training is key to good continence management. You may wish to nominate one staff member who has a special interest to act as a continence champion and a resource for other staff when needed.

As the home manager, attend a continence course yourself.

What is involved in continence planning?

Residents in care homes will have their own individual needs, but consider the following when planning continence care:

Personalised assessment of need for each resident who displays urinary symptoms or incontinence;

Community/district support from specialist services;

Regular management audits – improving care by acting on the findings without delay;

Policies and protocols that support the promotion of good continence care for residents.

2.2.3 Pressure ulcers – what you need to know as Registered Manager/Home Manager

This section, supplied by qualified nurse Rose Durack, covers the prevention and treatment of pressure ulcers, medication management, continence and the taking of obs (observations).

A pressure ulcer is damage to the skin and the deeper layer of tissue under the skin. This happens when pressure is applied to the same area of skin for a period of time and cuts off its blood supply. It is more likely to occur if a person has to spend a long time in a bed or chair. Pressure ulcers are sometimes called "bedsores" or "pressure sores". Areas vulnerable to pressure sores include the lower back and buttocks, and bony protruding areas, such as shoulders, hips, knees, heels, and ankles.

Without care, pressure ulcers can become very serious. They may cause pain, or mean a stay in hospital. Severe pressure ulcers can badly damage the muscle or bone underneath the skin, and can take a very long time to heal.

The definitions of pressure ulcer and categories (a rough guide):
- an open wound or blister – **a category two pressure ulcer;**
- a deep wound that reaches the deeper layers of the skin – **a category 3 pressure ulcer;**
- a very deep wound that may reach the muscle and bone – **a category 4 pressure ulcer.**

The language may be technical but, in basic terms, the Category 3 and 4 pressure ulcers are CQC reportable – they represent full-skin loss and full-tissue loss. Category 3 and 4 are serious wounds.

Ways to stop pressure ulcers from getting worse and helping them to heal include:
- applying special dressings that speed up the healing process and may help to relieve pressure;
- moving and regularly changing the person's position – repositioning – this can be up to every two hours;
- using specially-designed static foam mattresses or cushions, or dynamic mattresses and cushions that have a pump to provide a constant flow of air;
- providing a healthy, balanced diet;
- a procedure to clean the wound and remove damaged tissue (debridement).

Simply put, most pressure ulcers are preventable. They are caused by neglect or a lack of coordinated good practice and care. There may have been a neglect of: diet and hydration; repositioning the resident with a wound; treating the wound effectively; using equipment to help the wound heal and give the person relief. For these reasons, the registered manager would need to report it in to the CQC as serious neglect. Clearly, it's an area that needs coordination – but be aware that, if the skin breaks down, all the care home/nursing tools need to be used intelligently. These include: body mapping, skin inspections, effective personal care planning, the use of appropriate creams, pressure-relieving equipment and repositioning. All of this must be done with input from nurses/GPs /the tissue viability team, to stop the damage from progressing to a pressure sore. It's a complex area but hopefully the above gives you an idea!

Pressure ulcers/Know your residents:
Anyone living in a care home is at risk of developing a pressure ulcer. However, there will be certain residents at greater risk, and therefore the home manager should have oversight of such residents and their own particular risk factors.

Pressure ulcers/High risk factors:
The most obvious risk factors to be aware of are: restricted mobility, which may require assisting the resident with changing position on a frequent basis; any previous pressure ulcer; any current pressure ulcer; loss of sensation and feeling in parts of the body; skin that is dry and weak. Poor nutrition and dehydration are also key factors in the development of pressure ulcers.

Pressure ulcers/Getting a risk assessment/First six hours:
Depending on whether the role of registered manager is in a nursing or residential home, risk assessment will vary in terms of who carries it out and how it is done. For example, in a nursing home, a trained nurse should be able to carry out a risk assessment for anyone who moves in. Good practice dictates that the risk assessment should ideally be carried out within the first six hours of the person's moving in.

Pressure Ulcers/Managing the risk in a residential home:
In a residential home, if a person has one or more risk factors and they have been referred to a community nurse, it is wise to advise the nurse that the resident will require a risk assessment on their first visit, followed by a fully-documented plan of care for the staff within the care home. Depending on the local authority where the residential home is located, it may be that district nurses will visit the person in the home to apply clinical care as per the care plan.

If there is no previous or pending referral to a community nurse and there are concerns that the resident's skin integrity may be deteriorating, consider calling the GP, who can put you in touch with specialist services. Each local authority will have their own route to referral.

It may be that the GP or the community or district nurse is the first point of contact. Whoever it is, ensure that the correct contact details are documented in the home's protocol, explaining how and when to make a referral if concerns are raised with regard to potential development of pressure ulcers.

Pressure Ulcers and the care plan

There will need to be a care plan in place for anyone who has been assessed as being at high risk of developing a pressure ulcer. The care plan must be reviewed regularly; the home manager will need to audit it on a frequent basis, to ensure it is being adhered to. If it is not, the home manager must address this with members of staff with immediate effect. The home manager will need to address any reasons the plan is being neglected, by methods such as training, performance review and so forth – but it is the ultimate responsibility of the home manager to make sure that the care plan is delivered exactly as it is written, as there is no room for delay or error.

If the home manager is not familiar with pressure ulcer management, then it would be wise to access the relevant level of training in this area.

Pressure Ulcers and Safeguarding concerns:

If you do become aware of a pressure ulcer on a resident, then it is imperative that you as the home manager understand the local safeguarding policy and at what level it is expected that a person with a pressure ulcer should be safeguarded. Read the care home's in-house safeguarding policy and apply the principles within to ensure that best practice is carried out at all times.

2.2.4 Clinical Observations for care home managers

The broad sense of "observations" refers to the physical assessment of a patient, including the assessment of wounds and wound drains, intravenous therapy, pain and vital signs collection and specialised assessments, such as neurological observations.

What are vital signs?

Vital signs are used in the collection of clusters of physical measures, including pulse, temperature and blood pressure and respiration.

Why do care home staff take obs (observations)?

Observations are a useful tool to gauge a resident's/patient's health – especially for those who are very poorly. For nursing home residents, the observations for the patient/resident are taken regularly. If a resident deteriorates, the change in the observations reveals it. In some cases, the deterioration will lead to death. By capturing the timing and degree of change, it gives the nurse information to assess, informing their decision about what will be the best course of action. If it is serious, options will include calling for an ambulance, speaking to an on-call doctor, etc. In residential homes, the ambulances will be called more often, as there are no qualified clinicians on-site. In nursing homes, the nurse will take the vital signs and interpret these based on their clinical knowledge, with a deeper understanding about what may be occurring.

For nursing homes

Within Nursing homes, all nurses should know how to take and understand clinical observations and they should be up to date with any relevant clinical and mandatory training. It is the role of the nursing home manager to ensure that all nurses are competent and properly trained in taking accurate observations and making correct decisions and onward referrals based on findings.

For residential homes

In residential homes, staff will likely make general observations during the course of their work. They may notice a change in a resident's condition, such as: low fluid intake measures, low fluid output, loose bowels, high body temperatures, change in mood or behaviour. They may notice a change in skin integrity – such as red areas or bruising – while assisting with personal hygiene, and/or they may perceive a general deterioration overall.

Residential care home staff will also benefit from training in taking specific observations so that they understand the importance of observation and how to act upon any concerns. However, if the observation is of a clinical nature, such as the taking of blood pressure, then the appropriate course must be resourced in order to train the care assistant how to carry out such a task competently.

It is usually at this point that the advice of the resident's general practitioner is sought for ongoing intervention and care planning. Any of the above observations should also be reported to the care home manager so that he/she can take the appropriate action to ensure that future care and support is delivered.

2.2.5 What are the main responsibilities of nursing? (The fundamentals explained for the non-clinician!)

According to the trusted *Royal Marsden Manual of Clinical Nursing Procedures, Ninth Edition* (the long-established nurse specialist bible), nursing procedures are described as follows:

Part 1 **Managing the patient journey** – assessment and discharge, infection prevention and control.

Part 2 - **Supporting the patient with human functioning** – communication, elimination, moving and positioning, nutrition, fluid balance and blood transfusion, patient comfort and end-of-life care and respiratory care.

Part 3 - **Supporting the patient through the diagnostic process** – interpreting diagnostic tests, observations.

Part 4 - **Supporting the patient through treatment** – medicines management, perioperative care (pre-operation), wound management.

So, now you know!

3. General Management Responsibilities

3.1 Care Home Recruitment – how to get it right

Successful recruitment is the lifeblood of any care home. Actively recruiting new staff is essential to balance the high levels of staff turnover in social care. Factors may include the fact that it's shift work over seven days, often requiring weekend working. It also often involves late shifts – 2pm to 10pm, for example. For single parents with little support around childcare, these shift patterns can be impractical.

Ideally, a residential home wants to use zero agency workers, relying wholly on their own team of contracted carers and occasional workers (aka "bank" workers) to fill their shifts. In reality, most mid-to-large-size homes use a degree of agency workers on an occasional or regular basis. I recommend Neil Eastwood's book, *Saving Social Care*, as a reference to delve into this more deeply. There are several articles on the use of agency in care homes covered in my book, *Leadership Secrets for Care Home Managers*.

Care groups use different tools to recruit team members:

- **Company-managed recruitment job boards** – often these are not well-integrated into the most popular sites, e.g. www.indeed.co.uk. There is good reason for using an internal job board; in theory it saves money on expensive agencies. In practice, internal recruiters sometimes lack the level of contacts, skill and drive of financially-driven external recruiters (there are some excellent ones, too). The other limitation for internal recruiters is having no middleman to bring the two parties together.

- **Open days/banners** – can be good for attracting one or two staff members but, in my recent experience, with a buoyant job market in the care sector and many unfilled jobs at minimum-wage level, there needs to be more of an incentive.

More subtle issues that can compound the problem are:

- **Providers not adjusting the rate of pay for the local area, or having an uncompetitive level of benefits.** Though carers are not necessarily financially driven, often they will know who has better benefits. Sick pay is an important one, yet often omitted. The net result is that staff members work when they are ill and tend to run their health down over time, leading to higher sickness levels. This can be very counter-productive.

- **Lack of public transport to the home** – it all depends on the level of housing and depth of car ownership/demographics in the area. Sometimes it can work fine – for example, where staff members who own cars transport others who are on the same shift. In other instances, the lack of public transport can lead to long-term agency usage, which can, in turn, lead to quality/sustainability issues.

- **Reputation of the home/manager** – this has a significant bearing on recruitment. Everyone who makes contact with the home will form their own view of the home manager. In my experience, often carers/nurses who are very tough will rise to the top. Whilst their "firm but fair" management style is effective on some levels, there are other management approaches which would help engage a staff team. Home managers who have risen up through the ranks would benefit from being taught how their behaviours impact on the behaviours of the team. Skills for Care (the Government education and training partner to the CQC) does some great management training for care managers – worth a look: https://www.skillsforcare.org.uk/Home.aspx

Which is best – experienced staff or those new to care?

With so many new care homes being built, the care home labour market is expanding, making this an important concern for any home manager. My own experience of the pros and cons of each is detailed below:

Recruiting experienced staff:

The pros:

- They often have solid training, sometimes a Level 2 or 3 Diploma in Social Care.
- They are knowledgeable, safe and understand good practice.
- They cost little to train.
- They need little time to get up and running and be on the rota.

The cons:

- They can be burnt-out or institutionalised –
- When did they first learn about care?
- Have they adapted their practice as care standards have evolved?
- Are they leaving their current job due to problems at the care home?

It takes judgement and experience to decide whether an experienced staff member will be an asset or a liability. I always recruit based on emotional warmth (do they have any?) and on attitude – are they easy to talk to? Do they listen? Are they team players or moaners/complainers? Do they have a passion for care and making a difference, or do they just, "say the right thing?"

Recruiting staff members who are new to care:

The pros:

- They are a blank sheet of paper to a point with regard to culture/ethos – they will typically absorb what you say.
- They can be useful to bring some new perspective to a team.

The cons:

- They need a great deal of training to become competent – there are time and cost implications here.
- There is a greater churn for new staff – they may "try it out" and then leave, wasting valuable management and admin time.

All home managers have been burnt by recruiting staff new to care, who seemed engaged, made lots of promises, but left shortly after. It's a hazard and risk when recruiting from this profile of candidate. I've found that a very robust, structured induction during their first few weeks will help the more committed "new to care" staff settle. A degree of creativity and focus is needed to help these staff make a successful adjustment to their new work setting.

Interestingly, several CQC "Outstanding" rated providers I know have developed their capabilities to properly train and induct "new to care" staff to their ethos and standards. They actively prefer to take on staff who haven't worked in care before and introduce them to their values and ways.

3.2 Managing Finance (see also 'The Delicate Balance of Bed Occupancy versus Residents' Needs')

Fundamentals: Often the key numbers come from a detailed budget document prepared by accountants. It may be well-thought-through with input from those managing the service (realistic/achievable) or it may be a more simple affair where the owner/director simply states what they want to achieve in terms of occupancy (e.g. 100% occupancy all the time). The problem with an unachievable budget is that it is ignored and doesn't motivate managers to give their best.

The simplest way to look at managing finance for a care home is to consider four items:

1. the budget (the plan) for the year;
2. money in (income);
3. money out (expenditure);
4. the profit/loss (income - expenditure).

With a financial year starting in April 2019, the figures at the end of June 2019 will be April + May + June. If the home makes less than budget at the end of the financial year, it means they've "missed budget"; if they make more, they've "achieved budget with a surplus". During the year, if the home is not achieving budget, it is described as "not on budget".

The budget: The budget is a summary of the predicted money coming in (income) versus the money going out (expenditure). It is calculated for each calendar month with a tally for the end of the financial year. The difference between the two is the predicted profit (if income exceeds expenditure) or predicted loss (if expenditure exceeds income).

Income: This is based on a prediction of average room occupancy over the month and the price expected to be paid for those rooms.

Example: a care home has 10 beds and fees are £2,000 per bed per month:

If the home expects occupancy of nine people per month (average of 90% occupancy), the predicted income will be 9 x £2,000 per month = £18,000 total income each month. If the occupancy is predicted to be consistently nine all year, it means the predicted income will be £18,000 x 12 months = £360,000. If, historically, there is lower occupancy in December/January, the budget should reflect this. For physically vulnerable residents in poor health, a harsh winter can be especially difficult and in some cases will impact occupancy.

Private versus local authority/local authority plus "top-up": When a budget is built, the average price may be based on a combination of local authority-funded residents, plus some with a private top-up and others funded entirely privately. In this case, different rooms may have different prices (with a premium for ground floor, larger size, en suite, etc.). This needs to be factored into the budget.

Example: a care home has 10 rooms, with a mix of funding sources, as follows:

Four residents funded by the local authority at £500 each per week; one at £650 per week (£500 local authority-funded, plus family "top-up" of £150 per week); five fully-privately-funded at £1,000 per week.

This makes a total weekly income of £2,000 + £650 + £5,000 = £7,650 per week.

Expenditure: A detailed budget will predict costs across different areas of the home. The main budget lines to be aware of are staffing hours – across care, management, admin, activities, kitchen, laundry, agency, etc. There will be budgeted hours per department per week. There are also maintenance costs, catering costs (provisions) and agency costs. Staffing costs usually make up 45 to 65% of total expenditure. Of course there are many other costs, e.g. utilities, such as electric and gas, but these are not costs that can be managed a great deal, whereas managing staff hours against occupancy is something every home manager MUST do to stay financially viable.

The reason this is so crucial is that a budget will be set for a specific number of residents. So the budget might allocate £5 per day per resident. With 20 residents, the budget will be £100 per day. If you have only 10 residents, you need to spend £50, not £100. In short, the rest of the home needs to adjust accordingly. With only half the number of residents, there will be less laundry, less housekeeping, less demand for care, so there will need to be less spent in those areas. This is the essence of managing a care home budget. The skill is in *how* to do it. I offer some pointers below.

How to flex your staffing costs against occupancy: Staffing needs to be a balance of contracted hours and bank hours so that you can flex staff hours when you need to. A rule of thumb is to have around 70% of the care staff hours contracted and 30% picked up as extra shifts or bank shifts. That way, if occupancy reduces, costs can reduce accordingly. If contracted hours (people with contracts working regular hours) are 100% of the staffing budget, it will mean that, if you have 10 residents in a 20-bed home, you will still have to pay staff as if you had 20. The cumulative overspend will ruin the profit of a home and can cause the owner to run out of funds, which would in turn lead to a devastating emergency closure.

What to do if you're behind budget: If you're behind budget, you obviously need to increase the amount of money you make or minimise your costs. The options are: spend less, earn more – or both.

Spend less – this is about coming in under budget on your highest spending lines – maintenance, catering, staffing hours, agency costs. It's easy to spend less but the trick is to cut costs *whilst retaining a safe and well-managed home*. Of course, you can't any cut costs that might create risk for residents, e.g. by deliberately understaffing, which could lead to unsafe care.

Earn more – this may sound obvious, but this is about **earning more than is expected in the budget.** So if you have an occupancy budget for 18/20 beds and you had a month of only 16, the next month you will need 19/20 to catch up. The first and most important thing to know is how much you are short by and make a plan to catch up – e.g. in response to losing one privately-funded resident, you could look for either one privately-funded replacement or two local authority-funded residents to make up the shortfall.

Both – trying to tightly manage costs while attempting to raise income is hard but it will speed up getting out of the red(behind budget) into the black (being on track with the budget).

Managing staff hours/vacancies/use of agency and the budget: The key point here is that any critical staff vacancies – nurses, carers, seniors, etc. – lay the home open to the need for temporary labour in the form of agency staff. There are several issues with this when it comes to budget:

1. The cost of labour will be between 33% and 100% extra, if you pay for the shift on your payroll. It may include travel costs, too.

2. Regular use of agency staff can weaken the team by encouraging greater dependence on help from outside, thus lessening the motivation for team members to cover outstanding shifts from within.
3. Over time, care quality may be impacted as more and more staff come to work at the service who do not know the residents. This is not a comment on the quality of agency staff – which is variable and can of course be excellent – the key thing is that the staff don't know the residents and this lack of familiarity with residents and their individual needs multiplies risk over time.
4. An unexpected consequence of habitual agency staff usage is that existing staff may get burnout, as they carry more and more of the shift. This can result in more staff attrition – which, ironically, can lead to greater agency usage. Don't say I didn't warn you!

The key thing to remember is that the moment someone resigns you need to foresee an imminent gap in rota/possible agency usage. Equally, if you have any critical posts not filled, today is the day to push those roles, advertise, call those candidates, follow through, and get suitable interviews booked! You need to protect the home from resorting to agency; you need to protect your profit and loss statement; you need to deliver your budget. Habitual high agency usage (unless it's in the budget) will block you from achieving budget and once you get too far behind, it is very hard to draw back!

The difference between "profit" (private provider) versus "surplus" for a third-sector home: Some of the key differences in cost structure between charities versus private providers are that charities don't pay corporation tax. In some cases, they have boards of directors who are unpaid. This means their costs may be lower versus those of a private company, so, potentially, the service may be better value-for-money than a private operator. Charities also have a limit to what cash they keep, so if they make more than expected, it needs to be reinvested in the enterprise. This means that they are social enterprises, in being designed for sustainability as opposed to profit.

As a home manager, if you work in the third sector (charity), you will be expected to achieve your *surplus* (this term is used instead of "profit" within charitable organisations). Third-sector companies have to cover costs, salaries and building overheads – just the same as a private company. Third-sector operators expect managers to achieve budget/their surplus. Just because it is called a "charity", don't expect a lack of focus or vigilance about money! Every care service needs to be adequately financed. A key part of that is staying viable through effective financial management. The home manager is key!

3.3 The Importance of Audits

Quality audits are a line of defence against poor practice which can lead to non-compliant care and, ultimately, potential harm to residents. Audits need to be well designed and relevant for the service. Where there are gaps/weaknesses indentified in an audit, action needs to be taken swiftly and the home manager needs to be fully aware of the particulars.

Common errors in audits:
- An audit tool that's poorly designed/not suited to the service.
- An audit tool so comprehensive that it gets deployed only a few times a year as it takes too long to use. (One care provider I worked with made it so complex that it would take two or three days to complete – this is impractical and means audits will be less frequent, which increases risk.)
- Assigning audits to junior staff who don't understand the significance of items that need extra attention.
- A company culture where completing the document (box-ticking) is considered more important than actually auditing the service and taking remedial action.
- Under-resourcing the audit function – where audits are just copied from the month before. This shows a lack of rigour and exposes the home to risks.

- A lack of follow-through by the home manager – actions left/not dated or signed off.

The above points are regularly listed in CQC inspection reports where the rating is "requires improvement" or "inadequate". The key theme is, "It was picked up on in an audit and you didn't follow through".

The importance of the internal mock audit/the last CQC report

There are three types of full home quality audits that need to be taken especially seriously by the home manager:

1. The first is an audit by an external professional (a mock CQC audit). The actions identified should be completed and signed and dated in full. It should be taken seriously as it involves getting the home ready for a potential CQC inspection, ensuring the standards of the home meet the CQC key lines of enquiry (KLOEs): Is the service safe, effective, caring, well-led and responsive?

2. The second is an audit by the regional manager/director/quality lead employed directly by the operator of the care home. This is vital, as it maps the home against the standards and tools used by the provider to evidence good care. Failing to do this could be considered a breach of job performance as well as putting the home at risk. Audits are there to help the home manager run a good, safe service.

3. The third audit, and actually the most important, is the last CQC inspection. The home manager should take great care, providing written evidence to prove that the actions identified in the last CQC inspection have been taken into account, acted upon, and the new controls/standards maintained. The CQC will be very thorough in checking these matters when they visit; failure to do so will be considered a further breach, showing contempt for the CQC inspection. This in turn can lead to significant problems for the provider and home manager. The home manager and provider should take efforts to show a responsible and responsive approach to any matter raised by the CQC, to demonstrate that the home and service are well-managed.

3.4 Managing the Rota

Some key things to bear in mind:

1) **The staffing levels/allocation must cover the basic needs of the residents in your care** – that's a minimum of staff to cover care, laundry, housekeeping and catering. If there are absences on shift (weekends are usually the worst), these needs still need to be met regardless. In most homes, certain care staff will be experienced in providing cover for other areas too – the crucial two are kitchen and housekeeping.

2) **The rota needs to reflect a good skill-mix** – people put to work together need to have a sufficient depth of experience to cope with the demands of the area they are allocated to. If this doesn't happen, a more experienced staff member will carry the shift and may burn out/become resentful and eventually leave. This often happens in social care, especially when staff are regularly allocated to an area with a heavy workload. This can also amplify the risk of residents receiving poorly co-ordinated care.

For example:- there is a floor in a care home where a lot of physical work is needed, e.g. many residents require the assistance of two carers. If one of the staff members is inexperienced or has a slow work pace, then just meeting the minimum needs for the residents for that day – getting them up, washing, accessing the toilet, eating, drinking, getting changed – can be exhausting for the more experienced staff member.

3) **The live rota is a legally binding document to evidence staffing levels on a given day.** It can be used in a court of law in the event of a serious accident that may relate to low levels of staffing, and the registered manager will be held accountable.

For these reasons, the following good sense applies:

In summary: The rota needs to be a controlled document. It needs to be owned. Changes need to be authorised. Staff members must not be allowed to change it themselves; it must be managed through the deputy/duty/home manager, to ensure that the staffing cover arranged is safe and adequate and balances the needs of the team with the needs of the residents.

3.5 How to Manage the Night team in Residential Care

There are advantages for a care home to have care staff who only work nights. It means that the other care staff don't need to rotate their shift pattern from days to nights and back, which can be difficult. However, where a staff team have regular night staff, there is often a tension/rivalry between the night and day teams. This is usually based around the following assumptions:

A perception that, on some nights, the night team should do more – more cleaning, get more people up in the morning and lighten the workload for the incoming day shift.

The perception that days are harder and nights are easier

I worked nights in a care home for four years. I found the following: Working nights indefinitely has a bearing on an employee's sleep patterns and appetite. I found this can lead to brain fog, excessive eating and weight gain, among other health issues. Working nights is not easy on the body and mind. Staying up through 3am – 5am is *very* difficult.

Working on nights, with the absence of managerial support, is a very responsible position; there is a level of stress – needing to deal with all eventualities, having a small team to deal with any problems. I found the pressures and challenges in working nights to be different from those working days. You could say that the tensions between the two shifts are caused by a lack of understanding of the differences.

Important controls to manage quality of care at night

- Skills mix of team – making sure you have a strong team
- Regular staff supervisions
- Team meetings with home manager and acting on feedback from night staff.
- Sound recruitment and a thorough induction.

Unannounced night visits and audits by management (*see also section 3.3: 'The Importance of Audits'*)

These should be done regularly for two main reasons:
- As a deterrent to those who may be sleeping on shift.
- As evidence that the home manager is doing spot checks on care at night and performs audits of the service and building during the night.

The missing piece around quality on nights

Personally, I find it troubling that care homes will have a robust management presence in place during the day and then often no management presence at night. I think it is hard for carers who work nights, as they often miss out on regular guidance from the deputy/home manager. I would suggest developing a current senior on nights to become duty manager - nights. I would task them with specific responsibilities, give them extra training, an amended job description and, with it, an uplift in pay. It would be better for someone already working nights to lead the night shift. There are night-specific routines and habits of the residents which they will be better placed to understand. The lead on nights should also have input into care plans.

3.6 Meetings – daily versus weekly/monthly scheduled meet-ups

Daily meetings: Some hotel/hospital groups feel it's important to hold a daily meeting (sometimes called a "huddle", for example). The idea is to hear what different departments are doing and then ensure everyone is aligned for the work of the day. In my experience, the benefits of this are where there is a lot of activity that impacts on the staff teams – in that instance, coordination is key. However, in a small-to-mid-size care home with limited unique activity each day, I found these meetings to be of little value.

Weekly meetings: This is a useful format when:
- there are staff problems, either morale-based or behavioural;
- it is a fast-growing home;
- the home has a new manager.

The weekly format has the benefit of brevity – only talking about the last week. If you continue patiently, staff will usually begin to become confident over time about speaking up on issues.

Monthly meetings: Most care home groups will have a monthly meeting schedule, sometimes with a prescribed agenda.

For all of the above, the idea is that there should be regular meetings between the home manager and staff, residents and the various departments. The idea is good but forced meetings with little to say, or too many meetings, can lose sight of the intention – clear, effective leadership with good communication and a home manager who is listening and responding to the various people using, or working in/with the service. It is crucial to have good notes/minutes from these meetings and agreed action points which should be signed and dated before the next meeting. It is important for staff to see that the manager will take action on things raised at meetings as per "effective", "responsive" CQC key lines of enquiry.

3.7 Complaints and compliments

Compliments: This may seem obvious, but be sure to keep a log of compliments as evidence that the home is running well and having a positive impact on residents and families. There is a negative bias with care homes at times; capturing positive feedback is a great and authentic way of countering this negativity.

Complaints, concerns and queries: There is a distinction between complaints, concerns and queries. I see the significance as building – an unresolved query could be later cause for concern, which if left unchecked could then become a complaint. Queries should not be considered complaints. The CQC will want to see evidence of compliments and complaints, and especially a robust system for dealing with and learning from complaints.

You need to adhere to your policies and experience to weigh up the distinction so you are clear what constitutes a formal complaint, and what to record. Where possible, concerns, verbal complaints and queries should be dealt with immediately. Often, issues logged as formal complaints are in writing/email and explain a series of points or relate to a specific incidence where needs/expectations were not met. These will require a written response. Sometimes an investigation is appropriate, with a summary of findings.

Good practice is to use a form that shows what was done in response, with a follow-up and noting of lessons learnt, to prevent a recurrence. Complaints are a form of feedback and should be taken seriously and prioritised in a timely way. If you do not agree with a complainant's request or assessment of problems and proposed solution, you need to politely and objectively explain your reasons. Remember: the registered manager is there to meet the needs of the residents and listen to any other stakeholders with relevant information to achieve that end. You can never say you've got it all right; running a service is dynamic. We need to solicit and consider feedback and adapt continuously. Also see: www.lgo.org.uk (the Local Government and Social Care Ombudsman).

3.8 The Importance of Confidentiality

You might think that staff confidentiality towards patients/residents of a care home would be a given. Yet, in the rush of running a care home, there can be minor breaches in the spirit if not the practice of this principle of sound care home management. The guidelines of **GDPR***(General Data Protection Regulation) go some way to cover the need for patient/resident confidentiality but, like most law-driven compliance, they often lead to the creation of a series of rules which may not always meet the intention behind the legislation.

Regarding GDPR: ***From Department for Digital, Culture, Media and Sport Data Protection Act 2018, Factsheet – Overview:**

The Act:

- "Makes our data protection laws fit for the digital age when an ever increasing amount of data is being processed.
- Empowers people to take control of their data.
- Supports UK businesses and organisation through this change.
- Ensures that the UK is prepared for the future after we have left the EU."

This is robust around data but doesn't cover *verbal* indiscretions – direct or indirect. I guess what I'm referring to here is being mindful of sharing personal information about residents in the course of our day. Often, a care home can feel like a true community, with people mutually engaged and sharing everyday life – especially between relatives of residents. A family member may be curious as to where a resident they see every day has gone. Should the staff member divulge that they are in hospital and explain the cause? This is a dilemma – a balance between community spirit and openness, versus potential perceived intrusion in the sharing personal details.

My guiding principles are:

1) Consider what would happen in the outside world.

2) What would this person want – are they private or do they talk to everyone?

3) Who does the information belong to?

4) Concerning the person who wants to know/is expressing interest – do they have a right to this information?

Let's take a few real-life examples:

While I was working at a retirement village, a gentleman passed away.

A volunteer resident on reception wanted to know everything and felt that she had a right to this information. Considering the above principles:

The gent did not have a relationship with this receptionist – it's a village of 300 people.

In this instance, if you had 40 people living on a street, would someone go around each home and tell each person? Would they want that? If an undertaker came, would people who didn't know the family walk into the grounds and ask for an update? I believe they wouldn't dare, as, in most cases, it is considered to be private. That answered it for me.

While I was working at another care home, a gentleman resident was taken into hospital. A family member of another resident wanted to know where the gentleman was and what was wrong with him.

You could regard this as community interest or simply "being nosy". Do we say he has gone to hospital or what ailment he went in with?

Under the guiding principles detailed above, this lady didn't have a right to know, as she wasn't close to the gentleman. He was a private person. In such a case, the next of kin will be notified, as per the protocols for every care home. They will be given clear details as to what is happening, with feedback from the hospital. If someone doesn't have any next of kin, there may well be someone appointed with power of attorney (POA) for healthcare – that person will be updated. My sense of doing the right thing here was to let people know he'd gone to hospital, but to protect his privacy by supplying no further details.

Care home residents (especially those in later life) who are regularly admitted to hospital may feel embarrassed and not want to talk about their health conditions. They may also be afraid of death. Often, they will want to carry on as normal, getting back into their routine of everyday life at the home. From those staff close to them, they might appreciate some caring words or a reassuring hug.

To close here, I think we must remember to protect the personhood and dignity of every person living in a care home. It can be hard to keep in mind that, before they got here, they lived independently and had a plethora of life experiences. Though we call them "residents", they are simply people like us but older, often struggling to adjust to life on their own, within a community setting, and the resulting loss of independence. Based on my experiences of working across many care groups, I believe care homes do a great deal of good, far more than the media gives the sector recognition for!

4. Q & A

So you've read this guide, and you still have questions – here I cover some of the main queries that are likely to arise:

1. How can you research whether a care home is well run/good to work for? What should you look for?

Depending on how long the home has been established, the first place to look is their CQC inspection reports via the CQC website. Just type in the name of the home. You are looking for reports with a CQC rating of a minimum of "good", with no significant problems. The date of the report is important. If the rating is "requires improvement", that may be cause for concern. However, context is important; if the problems were highlighted a year ago and there has been no subsequent revisit from the CQC, it may suggest issues have settled. The historical reports are a useful barometer of the stability of the home.

Another place to look is the review site: www.carehome.co.uk. This site allows people to review the service. It is a good tool, but the provider can use it exclusively for marketing – i.e. soliciting only positive feedback – so the findings should be tempered with that in mind. However, if there are detailed and genuine-sounding relatives talking about how good and attentive the staff are, there is a strong possibility the feedback is genuine.

Other places to look online are employee review sites, e.g. the website glassdoor.com and other jobsites where they allow employees to rate the employer. Limitations here can be generalisations about jobs – carers may complain of long hours and low pay, for example, but this is not an issue exclusive to one care provider. It is still worth a look to compare the different ratings – at the very least, it is a benchmark.

Also consider how well a home is run/their culture as an employer. This is more subjective, with no absolutes, but the following may get you thinking objectively:

- How long has the home manager been there?
- Is there a churn with home managers? If more than a couple have left in the last two years, that's a sign of some difficulty. The same applies with the deputy role.
- Do they use many agency hours – especially carer hours? If they do, it may relate to problems with attrition/mask quality problems. There is not a definite link but high usage of agency carers over a long time often suggests a problem. (See also 3.2: 'Managing Finance – Managing staff hours'.)

Other general barometers are the level of engagement between the manager and the team:

- Do staff smile or look withdrawn/ignore the manager when you walk around?
- Is the home clean and fresh – does it seem that staff care about the environment?
- Does the food appear to be of a high standard –
- Are people living there enjoying themselves, smiling?
- Is there a comfortable familiarity between the staff and residents, or does it feel like an institution? Your instincts will pick up on this when you look around. If residents or staff seem bored or withdrawn, beware. It may still be a good place to work, but it may not be a happy place to work. It depends what is most important to you.

2. What does a deputy manager job entail? Are they registered with the CQC?

A deputy manager supports the home manager to keep the home running safely – usually in regard to staffing and resident care, together with any ad-hoc duties as per their individual split of work. This often includes support with audits, care plan reviews, etc., interviewing, holiday planning, return-to-work interviews and absence management.

The deputy manager's first priority is the actual care and well-being of those living in the service, and ensuring they are taking action on concerns or queries in a timely way and communicating clearly with those affected. For example, if a resident is moving towards passing away, there are various protocols in place regarding liaison with the doctor, nurse team, family, etc. These matters are time sensitive; any delay could have far-reaching consequences.

The second priority is staffing and the rota. The rota needs to be planned ahead to ensure there are sufficient staff on every day as per the occupancy and hours budget. It is important that staff have agreed those shifts. The planning of the rota needs to take into account the physical layout of the home, the levels of need for the residents in the different parts of the home and the levels of training and competence of the staff working together – "the staff mix". This is a key factor for having good care days – adequate and effective staffing. (See my earlier section on Managing levels of resident need and dependency with occupancy.)

After these two is everything else – holiday planning, sickness reviews, interviews, audits, supervisions, "being on the floor" – being visible and interacting with residents and families. This is work shared with the home manager and is dynamic according to the needs and priorities on the day and the needs of the many stakeholders who interact with those running a care home.

As per home managers' (*see Q & A no. 18, below*), deputies' salaries vary according to whether it is a private or charity home, nursing, residential or both, as well as based on location. In my experience, residential-only salaries are often £22k to £35k, with nursing-qualified deputies' salaries often ranging between £30k and £45k.

The deputy is not generally registered with the CQC, but instead supports the home manager, who is typically the registered manager.

Occasionally, a nurse-qualified deputy will be the registered manager for a nursing service.

3. What does a care co-ordinator role entail?

In my experience, a care co-ordinator is often someone who works in an administration/supervisory role within a home care provider. Different to a residential care provider (care home), they co-ordinate care calls to people's homes. These includes juggling visit times, hours budgets and service user needs with the carers available. A new customer brought onboard is referred to as a new "care package". A two-and-a-half-hour weekly care package could comprise care calls (visits) for five days per week, 30 minutes per day.

4. What does a unit manager/care manager role entail?

(Also read what a home manager does and what a deputy manager does, for a deeper context.) Where a very large home (say 150 beds) may have five separate buildings set out in a cluster, a unit manager/care manager will have operational responsibility for the 30 residents in one of the buildings. An 80-bed home could similarly be split into two units over two floors with the same structure. This role may include responsibility for care plans, residents, liaising with GPs and families. There may be an assigned staff team for that unit. It is usually a full-time role, with delegated responsibility from the home manager working in conjunction with the deputy. In some instances, there may be a unit manager for a nursing home, where the unit manager is an experienced care management professional (non-nurse).

5. What does a duty manager role/care team leader role entail?

This is different from the unit manager/care manager role, as it is often a post that is with a team supporting 24/7 cover, like a shift manager. The incumbent has defined managerial responsibility for their shift only.

6. What is a "nominated individual" (listed on a CQC report)?

The CQC regulations require that a person be nominated to act as their main point of contact for the service. The conditions for selecting this person are below (from the CQC website):

"The nominated individual must be employed as a director, manager or secretary of the organisation (i.e. they should be a senior person, with authority to speak on behalf of the organisation). They must also be in a position which carries responsibility for supervising the management of the carrying on of the regulated activity (i.e. they must be in a position to speak, authoritatively, on behalf of the organisation, about the way that the regulated activity is provided)."

Ideally that person should be separate from or senior to the registered manager, so that there is an escalation process if needed.

7. What is the difference between peripatetic managers, operations managers, regional managers and an operations director? Are they all registered with the CQC?

Firstly, let's explain about managerial levels:

- **Peripatetic (home) manager** – this is a temporary home-manager-level role for homes without a manager or experiencing difficulties whereby coaching is needed (for the home manager) or for extra support. The CQC can fine homes without a registered manager, so this role is important to provide continuity/direction for the home in the absence of a permanent home manager. By definition, then, it is an experienced home manager role. These managers rarely become the registered manager, as it is usually support provided for just a few weeks/months. The "peripatetic" manager will then travel on to their next posting.
- **Operations manager/regional manager/regional director** – this is a senior management role, overseeing home managers, usually for a region but it could be for a speciality, e.g. all elderly services. Sometimes the term "operational manager" refers to someone acting as a peripatetic manager (just to confuse things!). You can usually tell by the salary level. Organisations vary as to how much executive authority the operational/regional manager or director has. This varies from

setting budgets and strategy, with a line straight to the CEO, to a narrower level of influence within a more corporate-style, larger organisation.

- **Operations director** – covers all of operations with budget-setting responsibility, strategy, resource allocation, etc., and will be responsible to the CEO and board (if the provider has one). They are often responsible for overall CQC ratings, agency spend and clinical management – and are accountable regarding safeguarding, reporting on incidents and anything else relevant to the successful running of the care home/s.

What is significant is that, while all these roles have organisational responsibility, this is not CQC-defined levels of responsibility (unless they become the "nominated individual". This would often be taken by the operations director but, in some instances, it will be the CEO). This means the registered manager is accountable to the CQC *and* the organisation – whereas these individuals mentioned above are often *only* accountable to the organisation. (This can create conflicts/be interesting to navigate!)

8. **What does a home manager (registered manager) role entail in terms of responsibilities and tasks?**

The home manager is legally responsible and accountable to ensure the service is running in accordance with the various laws pertaining to running the home – primarily, regulation from the CQC under their inspections framework and, equally importantly, for the Health and Safety management of the building and all the safety regulations relating to it. The CQC regulation framework for good care consists of questions that are also called "key lines of enquiry" (known as KLOEs): "Is the service safe, caring, effective, well-led, responsive?" The CQC has defined ways of answering these questions and the expected standards in their guidelines. (See my earlier section on the CQC and KLOEs.)

The Home Manager is responsible to the provider within their employment contract to run the service as above and according to the measures of success they outline. It's a broad area but the items below cover the most crucial areas for this job:

Financial controls

The provision of safe, effective residential care can be expensive. It is a fine balancing act to manage the income and expenditure of the home to make a fair return or "surplus" (in the case of a charity).

The top three financial controls will always be:

1) Occupancy – how many beds are taken versus budget and what is the split between privately-paying residents and those who are publicly funded?

2) Hours – how many are being used versus budget? It needs to flex with occupancy.

3) The use of agency workers – If this course of action is being taken, is the home manager working toward ending it, and have they taken all other actions available, e.g. offered shifts out to everyone, half shifts for several staff, etc., before booking the agency staff?

Nursing cover

If the manager is running a nursing home, it is essential to have consistent nursing cover – this is a number-one priority; otherwise, the service is in breach of their CQC registration, and the residents are at risk of harm. This means there must always be an actual nurse in the building, 24/7, without exception.

Priority Areas

The priority areas for the home manager in the day-to-day running of the home are usually:

- Staff cover – are there enough adequately trained staff on shift at any one time and rostered (otherwise, the service could be unsafe).

- Safeguarding – are the safeguarding alerts being used properly? (This is to protect residents from risk of harm, while demonstrating openness and rigour in reviewing and acting upon what is found).

- The next priority is CQC notifications – the home manager is legally required to send through notifications to the CQC via email, using standard forms, regarding deaths, abuse and other specified matters. Are the notifications being used consistently and appropriately?

- Another major focus for the home manager is CQC inspection – is the home rated as at least "good" and is an inspection imminent – and are they prepared? The way to be ready is, firstly, to have an adequate system of audits and quality assurance within the governance of the provider. These need to be used consistently, with detailed and accessible record-keeping evidenced. The focus of the home manager is to regularly audit key areas to maintain quality assurance in the running of the home and to take action that is evidenced, based on the findings of the audits. The other consideration is to ensure any items raised in the last CQC inspection have been completed. Furthermore, any actions from other quality visits (either internal or external) must have been acted upon – showing the service is listening and responding to feedback.

There is a considerable body of good practice which home managers need to be aware of and practise in order to get a "good" rating and not be marked down. Some of this is very specific – e.g. are team meetings held consistently – where are the minutes? Are all reference checks done and DBS ("Disclosure and Barring Service" security checks) before starting – can you evidence it? Are fridge temperatures consistently taken – can you evidence it? There are many small details which need attending to and are considered markers of a good service by the regulator, their absence a consideration of a poorly-led service.

Lastly, the regulators will take a holistic view of the service – if a new resident comes into the service, was their care plan adequate for their needs? Are they being well-looked-after? Are they getting adequate fluids? Have they seen the GP – can you prove it? What diet are they on? What activities do they enjoy? Can you evidence you've provided it? If they had a fall, was there a follow-though? If they banged their head, was a protocol for head injuries followed? A well-run provider should have most/all of these protocols in place within their policies, procedures and agreed ways of working.

9. What are the differences between managing a smaller care home and a mid-to-large-size home?

Firstly, let's define these sizes – some care homes for specific specialities can have as few as five beds, so let's be clear: by small, I mean around 35 beds; medium: 36 to 55 beds; and large: 56 to 80 beds.

The key thing that changes with the size of the home is the size of the staff budget (hours). This has significance for the home manager. In the smaller services, it may be expected that the home manager work on the floor, providing care, giving out medication, and helping in any other way needed – from housekeeping to cooking. In some instances, if a staff member calls in sick, the manager may need to cover the shift themselves. This may be occasional or habitual if there is a staff vacancy – it is something to quietly explore at an interview. The same goes for nursing homes: if a nurse calls in sick and the manager is a nurse, the manager may be required to cover that shift. You can see how this needs to be well-managed, with clear expectations. The key thing for the home manager is to build capacity and flexibility into their staff team, to reduce their level of personal responsibility in covering shifts.

One other dynamic to consider is that, with managing a large home (as defined above), typically it is harder to get a CQC rating of "good" and above. Many of the services rated "outstanding" are smaller services, with 10-to-20 residents. This is more complex than it looks – to get a CQC rating of "good" or "outstanding" requires the feeling of "home", with the registered manager demonstrating a deep knowledge of their residents and team. When the inspector speaks to staff or residents, all conversations will need to reflect confidence in the service, and a responsive service, for a start. This is easier to achieve in a smaller service, where is there is a natural sense of connection with the manager, as you see them all the time. When the resident group and staff team get larger, the home manager assumes a greater sense of leadership and will likely be less hands-on. This requires a different profile of skills, including the ability to develop subordinates, to delegate and achieve outcomes through leading well, rather than by doing it all yourself.

10. What are the differences between working for a charity/private sector/corporate sector/small group/independent provider? Who is best to work for?

I guess the best way to start this one is to consider which set-up is best for *you*. There are a number of variables to reflect upon, which may help you to make your decision. If you've worked in the NHS a great deal, you may find the culture in a charity to be closer to what you're used to – less focus on "customers", with more focus on the values without a profit motive, and striving towards ideals of service with an ethical basis and a sense of equality. If you try working for a private company with a focus on business performance, you may find it hard to navigate – and you may be put off by their obsession with performance and results. If you've worked for a mid-to-large-size private company, you may be used to making things happen, execution and a focus on results and the customer; with that in mind, a charity may be a difficult transition.

In contrast to this is the small independent provider, i.e. one owner with just one or two homes. This brings a culture quite different from the two extremes above, for very specific reasons. In my experience, this encompasses a range of cultures, including amateur operators, where the home is like an extension of the family, very personal and comfortable but with unclear boundaries regarding roles and responsibilities. For some this can be comfortable; for others, the opposite. On the other side of the spectrum, you have small operators with a high level of knowledge and competence, who want the highest standards and will relinquish a degree of control and welcome the skills of the professional manager to help develop the service. Of course, there are all degrees in between. Only you can determine the best fit for you; you will feel it.

My only word of caution is, be wary if you are drawn to an operator closer to the first description: what can be difficult is where the provider expects you to do miracles, pays you well, and complains when you are not able to bring significant change. This is an impossible bind, as they may not understand their part in limiting how far the service can be developed. There is no right and wrong here, but clarifying expectations at the beginning and having a degree of awareness helps! The home manager cannot raise standards without being able to access some funds, be they for staff training or a partial refurbishment or acquiring better-calibre staff, electronic care systems, etc., or adequate staffing – this needs to be clear at the outset.

11. Is it better to go directly to an employer or through an agency? How do you make either work to your advantage?

This is a really interesting question and more complex than it looks. We need to start with understanding the value that agencies bring. In my experience, agencies come in three guises; let's call them Tier 1 to Tier 3.

Tier 1 – relationship-based, focused on good placements for the long term.

Tier 2 – partly relationship-based, but balanced with commercial interest – may have some practices which are not necessarily good/short cuts.

Tier 3 – will achieve placements at any cost – short-term view. Not always ethical.

Basically, an agency can work with good candidates and take time to find the right one for the right company – this is a slow-burn way of doing business, but effective over the long term. This is Tier 1 – quality focus. Conversely, a business can send CVs out to every job, whether agreed with the candidate or not, and may get lucky and get a candidate in/earn their 20% fee for very little work. In the end, it comes down to ethics and levels of professionalism. A good recruiter takes years to develop – they are highly valuable.

Back to the question, then: a reputable agency will represent you well, sell you into the role; they will do a good job of explaining your work history and motivation, connecting it to that organisation's mission and goals; they will pave the way for the employer to feel good about meeting you. They are like a dating coach, smoothing the way, helping both to connect. If you go directly to the company, there is no one to do this for you. If you have very good communication skills and sales skills, you may get on ok going directly and save the company money. If you don't have those two skills, often you are better off using an agency. Also, don't forget the value of a good recruiter: they often know the directors of many of the companies you want to get into. If they are good – Tier 1 or 2 – they can become a career coach for you, helping you to secure a good role that plays to your strengths and personality.

12. What is the difference between a residential home and a nursing home?

Good question! On one level, residential care is a term that means care in a permanent residential setting as opposed to care in the community for example. The other way the word is used is to make the distinction between a residential care home and a nursing home. They look the same and, to all intents and purposes they do the same thing (care for people needing support), but the levels of needs regarding the people they support (residents) and the manner in which they are cared for are subtly different.

A residential home is for people with a lower level of need/physical dependency than those living in a nursing home. Typically, this means those who can't safely continue to live at home. They tend to need some help with everyday tasks – washing, dressing, having food cooked for them, etc. – but their level of physical needs is low to moderate – they don't need to be under the continual supervision of a nurse. All residents living in a care home will be registered with a GP – staff will assist them to be seen by the GP as needed. If they have certain health conditions that need specialist support, a district nurse will visit them and provide support. The district nurse is not managed by the home manager but will feed back to staff in the home, and update care notes as required. This means there is a lighter level of clinical responsibility for a home manager managing a residential home versus a nursing home.

A nursing home is for people with a higher level of need (this is determined by a detailed assessment of their needs). Nursing beds often cost considerably more than residential beds, so a person is not deemed to need a nursing bed unless it is absolutely essential. Someone requiring nursing care may retain their sense of mobility or may be bedbound, but the significance is that they have a combination of needs which means that, for their safety, they need to be under the supervision of a qualified nurse. A nursing home is required by law to have a nurse on-site 24 hours per day/7 days per week to meet this obligation. Depending on the size of the home and the complexity of the needs of the existing residents, there may be several nurses on shift at any one time. With the current severe nursing shortage, in some homes this is creating significant problems; it can be that the quality of nurses available is low, which could compromise the service. It could mean an over-dependence on agency nurses, without continuity; this can introduce a higher level of risk to the residents and home manager. It can also cause the nursing home to be financially unsustainable.

The home manager *must* ensure the nursing staffing minimum is maintained, as it is reportable to the regulator if this is not met for even one shift. If there are nursing shortages in the home, it can be a significant ongoing challenge to maintain the high levels of clinical safety and good practice. The home manager is accountable and responsible for the well-being of all the residents in their care, so they have a vested interest in ensuring the nursing team is as stable as possible. This is something to consider when taking up a position in a nursing home. To keep a good reputation as a home manager (avoiding serious incidents where the home is at fault) requires the management and reduction of risk at all times. The non-clinical nursing home manager needs a nurse-qualified clinical lead to ensure that the nursing home residents are being managed in accordance with good practice and the law, and that the nurses are given proper training, supervision and support.

Nursing homes often have long-serving staff with deep experience. Sometimes there can be tension between senior care staff and nurses. Often, senior care staff have deeper experience around practical skills in patient care. They sometimes feel they are more skilled than the nurses; but, in my view, this is missing the point – the nurse is an accountable graduate medical professional, bound by very detailed and specific codes of conduct, as per their NMC/RCN registration. They ensure a person's care is suitably managing according to the law. Both sets of skills and backgrounds are needed. They strengthen each other.

13. What is a combined residential home with nursing?

It is common to have combined homes – that is, both residential beds *and* nursing beds. Often this could be 70% residential, with 30% nursing. There is good reason for this: in many instances, a resident will come in at a lower level of need (residential). Over time, they may decline and eventually become in need of a nursing bed. It is good for the families and the resident to not have to move home – this gives better continuity, as they can remain around staff and management who know them. However, as a home manager, it means you effectively have a small nursing home with a higher level of need to manage, in conjunction with the residential side which tends to run more smoothly as the residents there have a lower level of need/less complex conditions.

14. What about assisted living/retirement villages?

Assisted living/retirement villages are another hybrid concept that can work well. The key feature is that people retain their own homes, front door, etc., while living in some sort of group setting – e.g. 40-to-200 flats. There will be some degree of central provision. This could be in the form of a restaurant or on-site manager, extra safety features, a team of people available if necessary to assist with cooking, cleaning, plus care on call on a discrete/as-needed basis. The main benefit of the concept is that people retain their sense of independence and choice, but have help on hand when everyday living becomes too much. In my experience, this concept works well up to a certain level of need. There is a point where the depth of support in a care home outweighs the benefit of a person living on their own and struggling, just waiting for their carers to visit. There are several large operators of these retirement living apartments and they have been joined by other operators adding very large retirement villages over the past 15 years. These require large sites and very specific demographics to be financially viable. They won't appear in every town but they often work well in terms of resident well-being and satisfaction.

15. How much experience do you need to become a home manager?

There is no specific number of years' experience required in general – many adverts say "between two and five". In some geographical areas, there is an actual shortage of home managers. Some experienced home managers are not willing to commute for more than 40-minutes-to-an-hour each way, as working hours can be long. This can create opportunities for deputies and other professionals to step up to the role. I think it is helpful to consider the following:

Are you confident that you can fulfil the duties of the registered manager/home manager position, and can you back up this confidence with examples of where you have demonstrated you have the necessary skills, judgement and experience to meet these duties?

Are you likely to be competent to fulfil these duties, and is it likely that the CQC will give you the registration? See specific requirements from the Health and Social Care Act below:

Health and Social Care Act 2008 (Regulated Activities) Regulations 2014: Regulation 7

"The intention of this regulation is to ensure that people who use services have their needs met because the regulated activity is managed by an appropriate person. This is because providers who comply with the regulations will have a registered manager who:

- Is of good character.
- Is able to properly perform tasks that are intrinsic to their role.
- Has the necessary qualifications, competence, skills and experience to manage the regulated activity.
- Has supplied them with documents that confirm their suitability."

The level of rigour at the CQC interview process for registration is fairly high. In some instances, if a home manager has been previously registered, the interview may be less stringent. The first time a home manager gets confirmed as a registered manager is a career milestone and needs to be prepared for carefully, taken seriously – and celebrated! The interviewer is simply assessing someone against the brief above, and will ask as many questions as necessary to verify that the proposed candidate has the knowledge, aptitude and understanding to fulfil their legal responsibilities.

16. What qualifications do you need to be home manager?

This is an interesting point – adverts usually say "has NVQ Level 5 or RMA [Registered Manager's Award] or equivalent". Some may add: "...or is willing to work towards it".

There are two messages here – one is that, if you have the old qualification of the RMA, you are ok. The other talks about "equivalent", which is broad – this could be a nursing degree or similar. The CQC links this to the Skills for Care standards, which mainly recommend a Level 5 in Social Care Leadership (other qualifications which cover similar ground are accepted). In my experience of working for corporate-level care providers, if you don't have a Level 5 in Social Care Leadership, they sign you up to the course when you join and expect you to complete it within 12 months. Often, they are understanding when this isn't possible due to work pressures. It is quite hard to do a Level 5 in Social Care Leadership (foundation degree equivalent) when you are busy learning your new job. I completed my Level 5 in nine months but the average is 12-to-18 months. In my experience, the CQC is very focussed on you having a Level 5 because, on a practical level, it means you have been assessed against all the key requirements of the role. The moral of the story is fairly clear… If you don't have strong, relevant, equivalent-level qualifications or higher and you aspire to be a home manager, get your Level 5 now!

17. Once appointed as home manager, what is involved in registering with the CQC? Is there a risk in not being registered?

Once you are appointed as home manager, there is usually the condition that you acquire the registration – the provider is employing and paying you to become their "CQC Registered Manager". The provider can be fined if they do not have a registered manager, so they are keen to fill these posts. Their recruitment process (if well-designed and robust) will often have competency-based questions* for you to prove you have the knowledge and skills to do the job. This gives them a sense of confidence that the CQC will be likely to register you.

Questions that require you either to evidence your understanding or give examples that show you've demonstrated this skill/level of knowledge.

18. What are the salary expectations for a home manager post? What is the reason it varies so much?

The range is surprisingly broad – from around £25k to £30k per annum up to £80k. The highest I've personally heard is a package of £100k. One group I know says £120K-plus is possible due to a bonus structure!

Before you ask, "Who pays the most?"/"How do you get that £100k salary?" (both perfectly reasonable questions!), it may help to understand why there is such a broad range. There are many inter-related points that affect salaries. These include: resident fees, private/publicly-funded split of beds, number of actual beds, specialisms, risks, compliance/CQC rating and home manager attrition, company culture, company status (charity, private company or independent?). Let's explore a little further below.

Before we talk about what makes up the different salary ranges, one key point to remember is that the legal responsibilities are the same whether you are paid £28k or £120k. However, there will often be an implied level of expectation around skills and execution of strategies at different salary levels.

At the starter end of home manager salaries (£22 - £35k) can be smaller, domiciliary care providers, 30-60 unit assisted-living communities, and smaller homes of 5-35 beds; these may include more socially-funded residents, rather than private fee payers. This is sometimes due to the level of funding they receive and small profit margins, which will put the salary ranges at a certain level. Similar-size homes will have similar cost/price dynamics and that will determine the salary. Also, there is an element to salary around the levels of specific skills – the deeper the level of skills needed, the more structure, more cost and more fees, which all impact on salary levels.

Mid-range home manager salaries (£35k - £45k) can be mid-size homes – 30-50 beds for corporate or independents. Sometimes there is a bonus based on occupancy, e.g. if you have 50 beds and the provider wants an average occupancy rate of 95% for the month, that will an average occupancy of 47.5 beds occupied per month. This means some days it needs to be 49 to 50, while others it may go down to 45 as people leave, so a high average can be hard to achieve. The rule of thumb for good home managers is to aim for the bonus but don't count on it, as there are factors out of your control which may not allow you to achieve it. As the registered manager, the most important thing is to maintain the safety of the home, the quality of care and a good reputation by upholding the highest standards. Don't be tempted to drop your standards to hit a target. Your integrity and reputation are everything in this line of work!

High-end range for salaries (£46k - £75k basic, plus bonus). Mid-point for this salary range are many larger older people's services that average from 50 to 80 beds with a median of £50 - £55k give or take, depending on whether it is mainly private payers, a private company (more funding and a higher level of expectations regarding customer service can mean a higher set of leadership skills required in the home manager) or perhaps charity run, often with a higher proportion of socially-funded beds and therefore less fee income, meaning less money for salaries. Often, nursing homes can have higher home manager salaries than residential homes. Generally, nursing home beds are more expensive than residential-only beds.

There are, of course, exceptions to all of the above – this is a broad generalisation. Other factors can be:

- Struggling homes with a poor CQC rating may pay more, as there may be some risk to the new home manager. If several home managers have left, it can put the salary up as well for the same reason.
- Large homes have larger teams; you need to be a strong, robust individual to credibly run a team of 100+ staff.
- Large nursing homes with serious clinical problems may need a very experienced clinical manager and trouble-shooter – often with 20-to-30 years' experience. These individuals are in short supply and in many cases will not leave their current home, so it raises the salaries further.

The key thing is to find out the values of the owner/operations director/regional director. Find out how they support their managers, get a feel for the ethos and decide whether it is a good fit for you based on those criteria. Only accept a role you are confident you can succeed in. Reflect on all you've seen and heard and the culture you've observed. Above all, trust your instinct!

19. What is the difference between a "general manager" position and a "home manager"?

The "general manager" title is used interchangeably with the titles of "home manager" and "registered home manager". It is often used for larger care or nursing homes, where more beds require higher levels of carers and housekeeping staff, due to the staffing ratios. The management challenge of running a team of 30 people, with five-to-10 staff members on shift at any given time, versus a team of 120, with 25 people on shift, is quite different. The first is very hands-on; the second requires a greater emphasis on organisational and planning skills, delegation, managing priorities and relationship-building, with a degree of hands-on working woven in. It also often requires a different type of mindset – this is loosely termed "leadership". It is an additional skill to that of manager, though the two can overlap. The key quality of a leader is considered to be that people will follow them – follow their influence, direction and vision. As well as being experts in their area, they have some perception of where the service is now, an idea of where they want to take it – and, crucially, how to get there. They usually have some influencing skills. Effective leaders can usually communicate well (listen, absorb perspective and explain things clearly, tailoring messages to the audience). These leaders are generally attuned to the heartbeat of the team and, though they aren't led by the team, they do listen to them. It is a subtle difference that requires confidence and a rounded/mature outlook.

20. What is the difference between a "home manager" role and the "registered manager" position?

There is an important distinction and the overlap needs to be very clear:

A home manager position refers to the home manager responsibilities a person undertakes on behalf of an organisation as defined in their job description. The organisation provides the brief, recruits the person to do it and holds them accountable to perform the role in the manner outlined, with levels of governance and support. There will also be expectations – some of which are explicit (explained) and others of which are implicit (implied but not spoken). Implicit expectations may be to perform the tasks similarly to how the last manager or regional manager did them, for example. Explicit expectations might be specific tasks to be done regularly, or defined timeframes for completing time-sensitive tasks. Examples of this could include responding to resident incidents (e.g. a fall) and updating a tracking system or responding to safeguarding incidents in a timely, appropriate manner. This is the job holder's responsibility to the organisation.

A registered manager position is where a home manager (there are exceptions) becomes the registered manager for the service. This means that they apply to the regulator, the CQC (Care Quality Commission), to become the legally accountable registered manager. There is a raft of legislation outlining what this means – it is a serious legal responsibility and comes with considerable personal responsibility, due to the wording of the law. The CQC will determine if the applicant has the requisite skills, knowledge and understanding to fulfil these duties. They verify this through an interview where the interviewee needs to demonstrate they understand the requirements for a registered manager and how to fulfil them, with a working knowledge of the law, as applied to care homes. So, a registered manager has a legal duty to the CQC to run the home in a way that is compliant with their regulations *and* balance this with the organisational needs stated above, to fulfil the needs of their contracted position. The exceptions are where a deputy or clinical lead, or someone running another home in a group, may take the registration for the service if their skills or experience are stronger or better suited.

21. Can a generalist manager (non-nurse) secure a nursing home manager position?

Yes, they can. There are a number of reasons why a provider may be open to having a non-nurse lead a service. One that I have come across a couple of times is where a former nurse manager may have lacked general management skills or have underdeveloped leadership behaviours. As a consequence, they may have allowed the culture to become too hard (dictatorial) or too soft (the leaders are their friends/boundaries are blurred), which can be unsettling for the wider staff team. This can lead to friction, team factions and, ultimately, poor care outcomes. On that basis, the provider may feel a manager with deeper general management experience may be more helpful for the service.

It is a broad question to consider whether nurses make better home managers versus non-nurses (I explore this more fully below). It depends on both the individual and the specific needs of the service. In my experience, each person brings their relative strengths and perspectives to the role and often relies on others to balance their experience with complementary skills and perspectives. A non-nurse will often run a nursing home where there is a strong and dependable deputy/clinical lead to support them.

22. Who makes the best nursing home manager: a generalist or a nurse manager? (A generalist is not nursing trained but has more general management skills.)

In my experience, this question is part of a genuine, ongoing debate in UK care home leadership, where residents with nursing needs are involved. Chiefly, who leads best in this time of increased rigour, within the new regulator's framework (CQC)? Who has the most complete skills to a CQC rating of "good" or beyond?

I write as a generalist who has been challenged by some former clinical colleagues claiming that only a nurse/clinical manager can "really" do it. Clearly, there does need to be strong clinical leadership – but is there always an advantage in that person also being the home manager? I explore below.

I greatly respect my nurse colleagues for the level of responsibility and skill they possess. However, in my view, the skill of nursing is a profession in its own right, as is a head chef or a qualified facility management professional. Their jobs are organised with documentation, records, reporting protocols for legal and corporate governance and (in my experience) usually robust recruitment tools in place, to ensure duties and responsibilities are clearly understood and fulfilled. The home manager has oversight for reporting, standards and audits, and takes appropriate action as needed. They lead by example, listening and supporting.

For my part, I have been determined to show that the distinction between the two disciplines is overstated. For example, no one would say that a clinical manager can't learn the theories of management science and leadership. In the same way, there is no reason why a professional and skilled general manager cannot learn the fundamentals of the clinician.

In my own, small way, I have tested this. After 18 months, I have finished my Diploma in Clinical Science with a Higher Merit. Was it challenging? Yes! Understanding "peak flow, urticaria, oncogenic theory and target diastolic blood pressure" was like learning a foreign language to me! However, I discovered that the fundamentals are not so hard to grasp, as there is a sense and structure to this body of knowledge. In fact, fear was my greatest challenge over and beyond the technical complexity.

In conclusion, I think a better question is – how can we develop clinical home managers to strengthen their general management/leadership skills? Secondly, how can we develop the clinical knowledge of generalist home managers? While we consider this, I believe we need to respect the complementary strengths that each approach brings. In my view, there is no "perfect" care home manager, there are just you and me, learning, growing, doing our best every day and drawing on the teams around us. Inevitably, we'll all always be stronger in some things than others and, after all, running a home is a team effort. I am more comfortable to leave it at that.

5. Bonus Material!

Here are two articles which previously appeared on the nurses.co.uk job board. They cover how to win that new care home job or promotion, and how to make the most of the care home, once you've secured the role.

5.1 Secrets of Winning that New Care Job or Progression

First of all, it is worth reiterating a few secrets of good interviews and getting that job offer! For some, job interviews flow easily and well. Others really struggle with them. Wherever you are on this continuum, hopefully the following will help:

The Interview process is like dating – on the first date, both parties show their best side to create a positive first impression. Next, we get the conversation going, avoiding any blunders or causes of offence/words and gestures that may form a bad impression. If that goes well, we have further dates to build on this and explore whether there may be a lasting fit. There are courtesies and smiles. Everyone is well dressed. Both are on their best behaviour – it is artificial on some levels but necessarily so. As it is with dating, so it is with the interview process – the dynamics are fairly similar but with a key difference that the whole sorting/assessing process is condensed into a couple of meetings and conversations.

How to understand the dynamics of the interview

The employer won't tell you about the manager he or she has just laid off as s/he didn't like them or their temper! Nor will they tell you about anything untoward in the way they treated said manager. Instead, they'll have a big, reassuring smile, perfect manners (usually) and will talk about how you'll be joining a supportive, well-run organisation, and how it's a privilege to work there, etc. I'm not suggesting they're being dishonest, I'm simply making the point that this is a professional, structured meeting and that there are requirements around your behaviour, personal disclosure, and positioning that need to be adhered to for a successful first interview. They are presenting themselves professionally and expect the same from you. Ignore this at your peril!

Some do's and don'ts:

Don't badmouth your last employer or line manager. This is an absolute deal breaker, as the interviewer will presume you'd do the same to them. The interview may not end immediately, but the opportunity to undo that bad impression has. Instead, in advance, practise factually covering things that went wrong in a neutral, responsible way, so as not to put off the potential new employer. Remember, as I said before, the interview process is like a date – so keep it positive, factually accurate, and flowing. You are aiming to create a sense of rapport with the interviewer. Job offers are made when the interview went well and the rapport was good. It's not just correct answers that are needed, it's the emotion of the conversation that matters, too!

Do answer the question! It may sound obvious, but often, perhaps because of nerves, interviewees will not answer the question put to them. If you can't answer or have forgotten the question – say so, acknowledge it, ask to come back to it, but NEVER ignore the question!

Do turn up early – about 10 minutes early demonstrates good manners and reliability. This also gives you time to use the facilities, look around to get a feel for the place and watch the staff interacting, before you go in to the interview. It demonstrates that you are disciplined, organised and taking the interview seriously.

Do prepare some questions to ask at the end (it's so rare that people do). This sends a message to the potential employer: if the candidate is well-prepared for the interview, they will be well-prepared in the job! It is an example of positively presenting yourself.

Some examples of these questions could be:

- What's important for you in terms of this role?
- How would you describe the culture in this organisation/home?
- Is there any reason why you wouldn't feel comfortable to take me forward to the next stage?

- How did this role come up?
- How would you describe your management style, etc?

Do your prep! Again, this is so rare. Doing your interview preparation will make you stand out. Just because it is an entry level role – e.g. for a carer or housekeeping position – that doesn't mean prep isn't required and that you shouldn't take it seriously. If you make a good impression here, it may mark you out as a future senior, team leader, deputy manager, etc. It is a sign of a mature and responsible outlook. So few do it, so this could be your edge, this could make you stand out! In terms of preparation, at the very least I'd expect the candidate to research the organisation – find out whether it is private or a charity. I'd expect candidates to look at our website to understand the scope of the service/home – the number of bedrooms, etc. For more senior roles – activity coordinator, senior carer, deputy manager, home manager – I'd expect candidates to do a few web searches. Management candidates should ensure they've read the last CQC inspection report in detail.

Do ensure you can meet the requirements of the role It sounds silly, but it really is a waste of time for a carer to apply to be a home manager without having performed a comparable role or achieved some of the roles in between. The jump is too great. It is far more sensible to show some previous progressions – to senior carer, team leader, etc. – or demonstrate comparable management experience in another role. It is not just about getting the interview or the job offer, it's equally important to ensure you can do the job. Build your competence and confidence over time. Play the long game to achieve your career goals. There are no short cuts to excellence.

Want to step into the next role? Carer to senior? Senior to Unit Manager? Deputy to home manager? See tips below:

Before stepping up to your next role, if you want to get the odds to go in your favour, you will benefit from developing your knowledge, skills and experience to meet the additional requirements.

For example, if you want to be a senior carer, there is nothing stopping you from asking to become trained in some of their tasks. The clever thing is to do it for free, to help out. Over time, build it up your competence, always be willing to help. Then, when the role comes up, you will already have the required skills and experience. If you don't get the career break you are looking for, wait. If you feel you are being blocked, you may get that chance somewhere else. The key thing is to focus on getting the skills and experience first, then work on getting the career break. So many do it the wrong way round! If you were an employer, who would you give it to: the person who just keeps asking to be a senior, or the one who's always happy to help, always willing to do more, who is trained in so much more, and who can help with senior tasks? Exactly! In the process, you will become better at your job, more knowledgeable and more confident. You win, either way.

5.2 Five Tips On How To Improve Your Care Home

Tip 1: Make the home appealing

I'm obsessive about making care homes appealing. I'd like to explain why. How does it smell when you walk in? Fresh? Or a faint smell of urine? For me, that's unforgivable, unless there has been a recent, unpreventable accident. The reception area should be welcoming, clean, tidy, well laid out, with clear signage. Some places take it further, with fresh flowers and the smell of baked bread to make a first-class impression, like a premium hotel. These are nice touches, but rather than having a prescriptive set of do's and don'ts, it's better to form a set of principles around hospitality and thinking of the customer experience, reflecting the level of customer you wish to retain/attract. How you apply these principles is up to you.

The home needs to smell fresh

Firstly, the home should smell fresh at all times. To achieve this, the housekeeping team must be well managed and the building well maintained. The housekeeping team need to keep the carpets, floors, toilets and bathrooms, resident rooms, lounge and dining room all fresh, using the right materials and an efficient cleaning schedule. The other essential element to this is about continence management and the impact this has on furnishings and floorings.

There are naturally two parts to continence management – urinary and faecal incontinence. (See also 2.2.2: 'Continence Care: what you need to know as registered manager'.) The second is rarer but does happen as a complication – it can be brought on by stress in those with certain mental conditions and it can be an element of the later stages of dementia; it can also be in response to certain medications. Urinary incontinence is a lot more common and is managed by supporting people to access the toilet when they need to, as well as the use of continence products, often continence pads and pants. When these pads are removed by a resident and not replaced, there is a risk of their incontinence affecting the physical environment of the home. In some cases, this can be managed with chairs and sofas that can be wiped down, as well as some type of hard flooring. Before you think, *Oh that sounds great, this is what needs to be done* – how would you feel if you had to sit in hard, plastic-type seating all the time? It is not always welcoming. Comforting, warmer fabrics can form part of feeling at home and relaxing. In regards to hard flooring, whilst it is easier to keep clean, what about the increased risk of falls, and of those falls being tougher? Some older people are very prone to falls. If the hallway or their bedroom has hard flooring, it may mean they hurt themselves more when they fall. It all needs thinking through carefully, balancing risk with practicality.

The first experience of accessing the home needs to be positive

For me, first impressions are important. When someone comes by car to the facility, are the parking spaces clearly lined? Is it clear where visitors should park, versus staff and professionals? It is clear where the reception is or where you should sign in? Which book you should sign? Is there always a pen there? Is the foyer or reception area clean and appealing, well laid out and tidy? Does it have hand gel and a welcome sign? Is there useful information about the home when you first enter, including details of the manager or recourse if you are not happy? All these little details create a first impression. Is it clear what to do when you enter the home – press a buzzer, wait at reception? No one wants to get it wrong, be presumptive or feel uncomfortable. Make it clear and accessible.

Tip 2: Stand in the shoes of your residents every day

This may sound self-evident or obvious, but I don't apologise for including it. In my experience, it is very common for this to be lost as staff get into their own routine. Slowly and subtly, the service can shift to serve the needs of the staff, rather than those of the residents. The home manager needs to be ever vigilant. The same can happen in any organisation and is very common in healthcare. The home manager needs to keep talking about this. Talk about the customer experience and see every part of the experience of living there, through the eyes of the customer.

Here's an example. A few years ago, I worked for a premium branded home in the south east, where the owners wished to attract more self-funding, paying residents, but sadly the owners didn't fully understand the needs of this group of customers. The food budget was too low to serve these discerning top-tier private residents. At times, residents were given cheap powdered soup, minced low-quality fish on Fridays and no alcohol with their meals, which many were used to. They could not choose a cooked breakfast each day.

The owners couldn't understand what the issue was. They were keeping to a tight budget and managing costs, so they didn't see what the "problem" was. In my view, it was one of perspective. The owners were deciding what each private-pay resident wanted, without listening. They didn't understand the expectation of this social group. It was why so many respite stays did not become permanent residents. Had the owners stood in the shoes of the residents and eaten the food themselves, they wouldn't have come to the same conclusion. We need to remember that all elements of the service are put in place to meet the needs of those particular residents. We need to step away from the bias of our opinions and judgements. It is not about our wishes, preferences, or what we think they should have or want. We need to ask questions and listen, to know the residents' wishes and expectations. We need to give them the best we can, to challenge mediocrity and low standards wherever we come across them.

Tip 3: Set the tone around culture and behaviours

Culture is much talked about but not deeply understood by most. Here, I want to talk about it in the context of how to run a care home well (operationally sound, CQC compliant and commercially successful).

ALL visitors should FEEL welcome. This means positive eye contact from every staff member, and a warm welcome. All visitors should be acknowledged and find the staff team accessible. This sets a culture within the home that is inclusive and customer facing. We want all visitors to have a positive experience during their visit. For families with loved ones in the home, the relationships and kindness from the staff team reassure them that their loved ones are well cared for and the home is professionally run. This positive emotional interaction with the staff team also helps family members to cope with their own grief, difficult emotions and, in some cases, a sense of trauma that their mother or father is poorly/has dementia and is now living in a care home.

How does the management team respond when things go wrong? Does the manager ignore it? Use it as a stick to beat staff? Are they impartial or do they overlook it, when it involves one of their friends/a staff member they like? How the home manager responds here will play a crucial role in setting the behavioural norms, and establishing the patterns of interaction between staff and management. In time, these unspoken truths embody the feel and therefore culture of the home.

How is the culture amongst the staff team? Is it positive, engaged, valued for the most part, or the opposite? Does the home manager bend the rules for their favourites? That will weaken morale. It sends a message to the staff team that says "there's no point in what you do. It is all about who you know". Needless to say, that is a toxic message. There needs to be a kind, supportive approach toward staff by the home manager, with neutrality displayed at all times. All staff need to feel that good work will be acknowledged, and vice versa. Serious breaches of your policies should be dealt with in a proportionate and consistent way. Every significant action or warning by management needs to be considered as a message to the staff team.

For example, if mobile phone use is frowned upon, when a staff member is on shift seen using their phone instead of observing a vulnerable resident, the staff member could be seen to have neglected the resident and potentially put that person's safety at risk. Management needs to provide objective feedback to the staff member promptly. Repeatedly failing to act on this type of breach will eventually bring a sense of chaos and disorder to the home. Effective leadership entails focussing on and addressing significant breaches, with action that is proportionate to the risk/severity of that incident. It is also vital to be consistent, taking into account context and mitigating factors in how those breaches are responded to. As leaders with responsibility for the quality outcomes of the service, we need to take every opportunity to continually remind staff of good practice, so they avoid breaching the company policies. That way, when there is a serious breach, we can demonstrate that we've been supporting our team and championing good practice around care delivery.

We should put our primary focus on prevention and upskilling staff by coaching and training people so they perform better. It's tempting to focus on problem staff, but it should be done whilst nurturing your team. Many care home teams become broken and dysfunctional where a new manager becomes too harsh in meting out punishment/removing too many existing staff, which often will destabilise a service. It's all about balance: being fair and proportionate, focussing on good care and nurturing the talent and capability within your current team.

What behavioural standard do your senior carers adhere to? Seniors should be in post because they are the best within the team, promoted because of their work standards, ethics and respect from the team. Their work and behaviours should be excellent. They should be role models, highly trained, knowledgeable and competent. They should reflect the ethos of the home as defined by the registered home manager. They should be part of the management team, aligned to the home manager.

If this sounds like an ideal, a dream which no one achieves, you are right – and herein lies the problem in most homes. Most problem staff teams have their roots in overly dominant/anti-social staff members that have not been tackled or managed properly. Often these are senior carers in post with skill and knowledge deficits relative to their position. Without a deep understanding of how to manage people well and deal with interpersonal problems, they will often revert to undesirable management behaviours, including bullying. This is usually to maintain their sense of power and position, or to deal with staff not working in the way they want. This is often experienced as bullying by their team members, which harms the morale of the home and can cause mental health issues amongst staff. The misuse of power at work can be very damaging to a person's self-esteem. These senior carers need to be shown how to lead confidently and use supportive language to get work done without bullying.

Tip 4: Build a community with the right mix of residents

There are two levels of community I'm talking about here. The first level is the overall sense of community that is nurtured, celebrated with rituals, events, traditions and a depth of relationship, support and friendship between the staff and residents.

The second level is about you as the home manager needing to be deliberate and discerning in the specific mix of people that make up your community. Placements should continue on the basis that a person's needs are able to be met by the provider and that it works for both parties. In some cases, a person's needs change so much that, after adjustments have been made and different approaches tried, the placement is no longer adequately meeting their needs – or, in doing so, is having a serious, ongoing impact on the quality of life or the balance of residents. In these cases, the resident will need to be moved to another service which will better cater for their needs. Failing to do this can mean the majority being adversely affecting by one or two dominant individuals in the home.

It can be very hard, but we need to remember we are here to create a sense of home and community for vulnerable people who've often lost much in spending their final days in a care home. We need to try and make our homes nice places to live, with a sense of joy and happiness. We need to be clear about what mix of needs we are able to meet within the home and closely manage where residents' needs change, and manage that creatively and supportively. Only after all options are exhausted, with constructive meetings with other professionals and the family, should we acknowledge where a placement is no longer working. Managing the mix of people living in the home is key to running it well.

Tip 5: Have a sense of pride in your home

This is the something extra that great homes have. Some have it due to history, values (e.g. Royal British Legion homes – very well regarded), others have it due to an inspirational manager or leader. In these cases, there will be a strong team. Poor staff members will have been moved on or will have left voluntarily – the reputation will be strong. It will be well managed and staff will hear about the home and want to come and work there. I think we need to have a sense of pride in our service, we should stand for something, have standards, strive for the very best, to win and retain a good reputation. Recruit the best. Give our residents the best every day. A sense of pride is an attitude that everything matters and that our residents deserve the best every day. It's being vigilant to ensure standards are always adhered to and the service is run well, with a sense of joy, service, love and contribution: pride.

Index

Much of the material in this book is inter-related, which makes it hard to define the boundaries between topics. That is the reality of running a business, a staff team, and a CQC-regulated service. With that in mind, here is a brief index, so you can sort by subject as needed:

accidents	27-28
assessments	24-25
audits	49-50
Business Continuity Plan	20
care plans	25-27
category 2/3/4 pressure ulcer	34-37
complaints	54-55 & 61
compliments	54-55 & 61
confidentiality	55-57
continence	30-34 & 87-88
CQC inspection reports	13-15, 50 & 59
CQC notifications	15-16 & 66
culture and behaviours	89-92
dependency	23-25
discretion (confidentiality)	55-57
finance (managing)	44-49
fire safety	19-20
first 6 hours after admission	36
health and safety	18-22
housekeeping	22, 46, 51, 67, 77 (Q&A) 85 & 87
incidents	27-28
incontinence	30-34 & 87-88
infection control	19

interviews (having)	83-85
job-boards	41
kitchen	22, 46, 51
KLOEs	13-15
managing finance	44-49
meds management	28-30
meetings	52 & 53-54
nights	52-53
nursing (responsibilities)	38-39
occupancy	23-24
open days	41
PEEPs	20
person centred	88-89
personal pride	93
pressure ulcers	34-37
queries	54-55 & 61
recruitment	41-44
resident mix	92
risk assessment	22, 26 & 36
rota	51-52
Safe storage of food and beverage	20-21
safe storage of medication	21
safeguarding	16-18
Six Rights of Medication	29
staff costs	47-48
urine smell in home	87-88
vital signs (obs)	37-38

A Final Note from the Author

Thank you for reading this book. I hope you've found it helpful. If you'd like to know more, there are four ways you can interact with me:

For care providers: I often get enquiries about using extracts from my work for good practice guides for mid-to-large-size care groups. I am happy to explore this with you. You can email me: **liam@carehomeleadership.org**.

For individuals:

- **Access the podcast** – Simply Google "Care Quality – Meet the Leaders & Innovators", and you will find the podcast on all major platforms. As of 12.07.20, there are 13 episodes.
- **Read my other books**. My first was *Management Development for Care Home Managers* (2016). The second, *Leadership Secrets for Care Home Managers* (2018), incorporates the text from the first book and can be bought on Amazon. The first book is available on Audible, too.
- **If you'd like help in preparing for a care home manager interview** – If I have time, I can provide a brief coaching session to help you prepare as well as possible to maximise your chances.
  Email me: **liam@carehomeleadership.org**.

I also recommend the following website as an excellent source of information: www.skillsforcare.org.uk.

Liam Palmer

Printed in Great Britain
by Amazon